Anti-infective Guidelines for Community-acquired Infections

2013 Edition

Anti-infective Review Panel

> *Peer-reviewed*

> *Evidence-based*

> *User-friendly*

See www.mumshealth.com for information on updates, iPhone apps and CME

This independent initiative is supported entirely through purchases of the guideline. All proceeds are directed to maintaining and updating the guidelines.

Comment sheets are provided at the end of the document and at the website.

Check the website for updates and full citations.

To purchase copies visit the website, email, call or fax:

MUMS GUIDELINES

**Tel: 416-597-6867 or toll free: 1-877-876-4580
Fax: 416-597-8574 or toll free: 1-866-540-1847
E-mail: guidelines@mumshealth.com**

www.mumshealth.com

Check the website or page 112 for CME activities and Community Antimicrobial Stewardship Initiatives such as: PAACT (PArtners for Appropriate Community Therapy)

Library and Archives Canada Cataloguing in Publication

Anti-infective guidelines for community-acquired infections / Anti-infective Review Panel. -- 2013 ed.

Includes bibliographical references.
ISBN 978-1-894332-14-9

1. Antibiotics--Therapeutic use. 2. Community-acquired infections--Treatment.
3. Communicable diseases--Treatment. 4. Family medicine. 5. Primary care (Medicine).
I. Anti-infective Review Panel II. MUMS Guideline Clearinghouse

RC111.A58 2013   616.9'06   C2013-901649-X

While great effort has been taken to assure the accuracy of the information, the Review Panel, publisher, printer and others contributing to the preparation of this document cannot accept liability for errors, omissions or any consequences arising from the use of the information. Since this document is not intended to replace other information, physicians are urged to consult the manufacturer's and other available drug information literature before prescribing.

Citation: Anti-infective Review Panel. Anti-infective guidelines for community-acquired infections. Toronto: MUMS Guideline Clearinghouse; 2013.

Table of Contents

Continued ...

Genitourinary Infections

Central Nervous System Infections

Gastrointestinal Infections

Prophylaxis

Appendices

References: For full citations see www.mumshealth.com

THE ANTI-INFECTIVE REVIEW PANEL

The panel represents a mix of health professionals with expertise in several fields, and who practise in a variety of clinical settings. Their names, areas of expertise and places of practice are listed below.

Dr. Steve Arshinoff
Ophthalmology
University of Toronto
Toronto, ON

Dr. Elise Balaisis
Family Medicine
Vancouver, BC

Dr. Andrew Braude
Respiratory Medicine
North York General Hospital
Willowdale, ON

Dr. Charles Chan
Respiratory Medicine
University Health Network
Toronto, ON

Dr. John Conly
Infectious Diseases
University of Calgary
Calgary, AB

Dr. Gerald Evans
Infectious Diseases
Kingston General Hospital
Kingston, ON

Dr. Geordie Fallis
Family Medicine
Don Mills, ON

Dr. David Greenberg
Family Medicine
Toronto, ON

Dr. John Jordan
Family Medicine
London, ON

Dr. Alan Kaplan
Family & Emergency Medicine
Brampton, ON

Dr. Tessa Laubscher
Family Medicine
Saskatoon, SK

Dr. Donald Low
Microbiology
Mount Sinai Hospital
Toronto, ON

Dr. Frances Mah
Ophthalmology
University of Pittsburgh
Pittsburgh, USA

Dr. Lionel Mandell
Infectious Diseases
McMaster University
Hamilton, ON

Dr. Frank Martino
Family & Emergency Medicine
Brampton, ON

Dr. Allison McGeer
Microbiology
Mount Sinai Hospital
Toronto, ON

Dr. Warren McIsaac
Family Medicine
Toronto, ON

Dr. James Meuser
Family Medicine
Toronto, ON

Dr. Curtis Nickel
Urology
Kingston, ON

Dr. Lindsay Nicolle
Infectious Diseases
Health Sciences Centre
Winnipeg, MB

Dr. Ross Pennie
Infectious Diseases
Brantford General Hospital
Brantford, ON

Monique Pitre, BScPhm
Clinical Pharmacist
University Health Network
Toronto, ON

Dr. Ross Prince
Urology
Oakville, ON

Dr. Jean-Claude Quintal
Family Medicine
Dalhousie, NB

Dr. Walter Rosser
Family Medicine
Queen's University
Kingston, ON

Dr. John Rutka
ENT
University Health Network
Toronto, ON

Dr. Marina Salvadori
Pediatric Infectious Diseases
Children's Hospital
London, ON

Dr. Fiona Smaill
Infectious Diseases
McMaster University
Hamilton, ON

Dr. John Stewart
Family Medicine
Port Perry, ON

Dr. Irene Turpie
Geriatrics
Hamilton, ON

Dr. Serena Verma
Family Medicine
Vancouver, BC

Charlene Welsh
Nurse Practitioner
Toronto, ON

Dr. Kevin Woo
Wound Healing Centre
Women's Collge Hospital
Toronto, ON

Dr. George Zhanel
Medical Microbiology
Winnipeg, MB

Scientific Editors:
Laurie Dunn, MSc, BScPhm
John Pilla MSc, BScPhm

Norman Dewhurst, Pharm D
Saadia Fazil, PharmD
Jon Hunchuk, PharmD
Harris Iacovides, Pharm D
Neal Irfan, PharmD
So-Hee Kang, Pharm D
Monica Lee, PharmD
Mohammed Mahdi, PharmD (C)
Damen Man, PharmD
Bekkyann Persaud, BSc (Hons)
Vishal Pua, BSc (Hons)
Marc Riachi, BSc Phm
An Sada, PharmD
Matthew Swankhuizen, PharmD (C)
Rosanne Thalakada, PharmD (C)
Jeffrey Wong, BScPhm
Lisa Zhu, PharmD

GUIDELINE REVIEWERS

Many thanks to the individuals below who have been part of our extensive and continual review process over the course of the past 20 years. We greatly appreciate your support.

Alberta

Maria & Zieten Basztenda
Community Pharmacy

Dr. Tom Marrie
Infectious Diseases

Dr. Catherine McKenna
Family Medicine

Dr. Peter Norton
Family Medicine

Dr. Pieter Oosthuizen
Family and Emergency Medicine

Dr. Barbara Romanowski
Infectious Diseases

Dr. Stephen Shafran
Infectious Diseases

Dr. Dilip Shamanna
Family Medicine

British Columbia

Dr. Richard Bachand
Clinical Pharmacy

Dr. James R. Busser
Internal Medicine

Dr. Allison Ferg
Family Medicine

Dr. Vincent Ho
Dermatology

Dr. Robert D. Levy
Respiratory Medicine

Dr. David M. Patrick
Infectious Diseases

Thomas Tse
Pharmacy

Dr. H. C. George Wong
Allergy/
Clinical Immunology

Manitoba

Dr. Robert Ariano
Clinical Pharmacy

Dr. John M. Embil
Infectious Diseases

Dr. Alfred S. Gin
Clinical Pharmacy

Dr. Peter Kirk
Family Medicine

Dr. C. R. Norman
Family Medicine

Dr. George Zhanel
Medical Microbiology

New Brunswick

Dr. Hamad Khatib
Family Medicine

Newfoundland

Dr. Jim Hutchinson
Infectious Diseases/
Medical Microbiology

Nova Scotia

Dr. Roger Thomas
Family Medicine

Dr. Ambrose Lee
Emergency Medicine

Dr. Andrew McIvor
Respiratory Medicine

Dr. Bruce McLeod
Emergency Medicine

Dr. Nancy Murphy
Family Medicine

Dr. Kathryn Slayter
Clinical Pharmacy

North West Territories

Dr. Wendy Hamilton
Family Medicine

Ontario

Dr. Deena Ages
Family Medicine

Dr. David A. Apramian
Family Medicine

Dr. N. Appekar
Family Medicine

Zubin Austin
Professor - Therapeutics
(Pharmacy Practice)

Dr. Meyer Balter
Respiratory Medicine

Dr. Harry Birman
Respiratory Medicine

Dr. W. Black
Family Medicine

Dr. Christine Bradley
Respiratory Medicine

Dr. Hartley Bressler
Family Medicine/
Chiropractor

Dr. Janis Browne
Family Medicine

Dr. Nick Busing
Family Medicine

Dr. John Carlisle
College of Physicians and
Surgeons

Nadya Chorostil
Pharmacist

Dr. Douglas Clark
Family Medicine

Dr. Aileen Comerton
Family Medicine

Beth Cowper-Fung
Nurse Practitioner

Dr. Alan Davis
Family and Emergency Medicine

Kathie Donnelly-Parent
Primary Health

Sylvain Duchaine
General Practice

Dr. A. Duic
Paediatrics

Dr. Nihad Fahmi
Geriatric General Surgery

Dr. A.J. Fegelman
Family Medicine

Dr William Feldman
Paediatrics

Sue Finnie
Nurse Practitioner

Brent Fraser
Pharmacy

Dr. Tom Freeman
Family Medicine

Dr. Jacob Friedberg
Paediatric Otolaryngology

Dr. Allison Geffer
Family Medicine

Mary Gordon
Community Health - STDs

Dr. Leonard Grbac
Family Medicine

Bella Grunfeld
Nurse Practitioner

Dr. Richard Haber
Dermatology

Dr. Karl Hartwick
Family Medicine

Dr. Michael Hawke
ENT

Dr. Brian Haynes
Internal Medicine

Dr. Robert Heyes
Family Medicine

Dr. Sheila Horen
Family Medicine

Carol Hobbs
Nurse Practitioner

Dr. Peter Hopkins
Emergency Medicine

Dr. H. Hotz
Paediatrics

Dr Richard Johnston
Obstetrics & Gynaecology

Dr. John Jordan
Family Medicine

Dr. Jay Keystone
Tropical Disease Medicine

Dr. Caroline Knight
Family Medicine

Deanna Laws
College of Pharmacy

Dr. Isra Levy
Family Medicine

Dr. Marie Louie
Infectious Disease

Dr. David MacPherson
Family Medicine

Dr. Bernard Marlow
Family Medicine

Dr. Frank Martino
Family Medicine

Dr. Warren McIsaac
Family Medicine

Dr. Shelagh McRae
Family Medicine

Dr. James McSherry
Family Medicine

Dr. J. Curtis Nickel
Urology

Colleen Nisbet
Public Health

Dr. Pete Nodl
Family Medicine

Christine Ough
Pharmacy

Dr. Alice Parker
Family Medicine

Sanjay Patel
Community Pharmacy

Dr. Rupa Patel
Family Medicine

Dr. Nick Pimlott
Family Medicine

Dr. Anita Rachlis
Infectious Diseases

Dr. Sidney B. Radomski
Urology

Dr. Neil V. Rau
Infectious Diseases

Chris Ritskes
Pharmacy

Dr Stephen Roedde
Emergency Medicine

Dr. Cheryl Rosen
Dermatology

Dr. Morris Rotbard
Family Medicine

Gerald Rotenberg
Pharmaceutical Consultant

Dr. A. Shayan
Family Medicine

Dr. David Schramm
Otolaryngologist/
Otologist

Dr. Sandra Tailor
Clinical Pharmacy

Dr. Philip Vandewalle
Family Medicine/Professor

Dr. Chad Wallace
Community Pharmacy

Dr. Shayna Watson
Family Medicine - Rural

Dr. William Watson
Family Medicine

Dr. Gordon Watt
Emergency Medicine/
Occupational Health

Sandra Winkelbauer
Drug Information

Patrick Wong
Community Pharmacy

Dr. Thomas Wong
Family Medicine

Dr. L. Young
Family Medicine

Melanie Zabawa
Pharmacy

Dr. Dick Zoutman
Infectious Diseases

Quebec

Dr. Jacques Allard
Geriatric Medicine

Dr. Jocelyne Bonin
Family Medicine

Dr. Francine Borduas
Family Medicine

Dr. Alex Ferenczy
Pathology/Gynecology

Dr. Diane Jolicoeur
Family Medicine

Dr. Louise Nasmith
Family Medicine

Dr. Paolo Renzi
Respiratory Medicine

Dr. Karl Weiss
Infectious Diseases

Saskatchewan

Dr. Tessa Laubscher
Family Medicine

Dr. Crystal Littwin
Family Medicine

Dr. J. Stewart McMillan
Family Medicine

Paul Melnyk
Drug Information

Loren Regier
Clinical Pharmacy

Dr. Yvonne Shevchuk
Clinical Pharmacy

Dr. Gill White
Family Medicine

Yellowknife

Dr. C. Breitkreutz
Family Medicine

Scientific staff, previous editions:

Erika Buckwald
Elaine Cheng, PharmD
Roger Cheng, PharmD
Cory Cowan, PharmD
Elizabeth Kozyra, PharmD
Lisa Kwok, PharmD
Derek Lee, PharmD
Marianna Leung, PharmD
Mova Leung, PharmD
Bob MacLean, PharmD
Katrina Mulherin, PharmD
Laura Murphy, PharmD
Andrea Narducci, PharmD
Nastaran Ostad, PharmD
Mark Pasetka, PharmD
Amita Patel, PharmD
Suzanne Singh, PharmD
Mary Vilay, PharmD
Stella Yoo, PharmD

PREFACE

Nearly twenty years have passed since the release of the first edition of the *Anti-infective Guidelines for Community-acquired Infections*. We have continued to receive hundreds of positive comments from practitioners across Canada and internationally regarding its content and user-friendliness. We sincerely thank you for your ongoing support.

The rise of drug-resistant organisms has made it difficult to know the specific place in therapy of each anti-infective in the treatment of infectious diseases. To make the job easier, the Anti-infective Review Panel, an independent body composed of family physicians, infectious disease specialists, pharmacists and nurse practitioners, has developed general guidelines to assist in the process of selecting which, if any, anti-infective therapy is required.

Physicians generally base therapeutic decisions on their clinical experience, specific patient factors, laboratory results, available medical information plus advice from colleagues and experts. These guidelines are intended to meet the needs of busy family practitioners for concise, relevant advice when initially selecting empiric antimicrobial therapy for common community infections.

The panel believes these guidelines, which have been updated with the latest evidence on anti-infectives and feedback from hundreds of health professionals, can be a complementary, educational tool to promote the most appropriate use of medications and the best practice of medicine. However, they are not intended to replace a physician's judgment and, in addition, are not to be used solely as a tool for cost-containment strategies.

GUIDELINE DEVELOPMENT PROCESS

The development process, known as the ***PGD (Peer-reviewed Guideline Development) Process***, is outlined in Figure 1 on the following page. This unique, inclusive and transparent process helps assure the guideline is evidence-based and relevant to daily community practice. An extensive literature review combined with comments from the previous edition (received individually or at a PArtners for Appropriate Community Therapy (PAACT) CME session) were initially used to create the revised guideline draft. This draft was reviewed by the panel and then redrafted. The draft document was circulated for peer-review by medical practitioners (generalists and specialists), academia, government, associations and the pharmaceutical industry. Their suggestions were reviewed, without revealing the identity of the reviewers to the panel, and the document was redrafted.

This PGD Process combined with the balanced composition of the panel (i.e., infectious disease specialists, family physicians, nurse practitioners and pharmacists) was instrumental in limiting the many types of bias, including competing or conflicting interests. Hence, panel members were not asked to declare any existing or potential competing interests, financial or otherwise.

The production of reputable, clinical guidelines is a continual process requiring the active, ongoing participation of front line practitioners. The panel strongly encourages you to submit any suggestions on the comment page at the back of the guideline or by email to guidelines@mumshealth.com. They will be thoroughly reviewed prior to publication of the next edition. We look forward to receiving your continuing support and participation.

ACKNOWLEDGEMENTS

We wish to acknowledge the assistance and expertise offered by the numerous clinicians who reviewed the document and provided invaluable input. Many thanks to Bekkyann Persaud and Nathan Pilla for their assistance in desktop publishing and to Matthew Eastman for fielding inquiries.

Figure 1. The Peer-reviewed Guideline Development (PGD) Process

Extensive review of existing literature, guidelines and comments from previous edition

↓

Preparation of a working background document for review by the Anti-infective Review Panel

↓

Redraft of guidelines circulated for <u>peer review</u> and feedback

↓

Peer reviewers' comments presented to the Anti-infective Review Panel. To ensure impartial assessment, the source (name and affiliation) of the comments was not revealed

↓

Guidelines redrafted with modifications and circulated to Panel for final approval

↓

Guidelines printed and disseminated to health practitioners, etc.

↓

Guideline implemented with multi-dimensional strategies and followed with evaluation

↓

Guidelines revised regularly based on comments from users and the emergence of new evidence. For up-dates see: *www.mumshealth.com*

USE OF THE GUIDELINES

General

Selecting the appropriate antibiotic involves consideration of the location of the infection and clinical diagnosis, sensitivity patterns of possible organisms involved, host factors, treatment setting and cost (when efficacy and toxicity issues are equivalent). Where possible an effort has been made to provide specific drug choices, rather than broad classes, since this is more practical and useful to primary care practitioners.

The first, second and third line choices of antibiotics in these guidelines have been carefully selected based on spectrum of activity, anticipated efficacy, safety, previous clinical experience and resistance patterns. Drugs listed within the first, second or third line categories may be considered equally efficacious and any one within the category can be considered as a therapeutic choice. Many of the second and third line agents may be as effective as first line agents. They have been listed as alternatives because of considerations such as resistance, intolerance, spectrum of activity, potential noncompliance and cost. Drugs are generally listed in order from least to most expensive, however therapeutic classes have been grouped together (e.g., cephalosporins, macrolides, etc.). In general, older antibiotics (generally more narrow spectrums) should not be replaced with newer drugs unless efficacy is substantially improved, toxicity is reduced or they are more cost effective.

References throughout the document use the primary author's last name and year of publication (Doe 2013). **Complete references are available at www.mumshealth.com.**

Dosage

An effort has been made to suggest oral products, wherever feasible, and the products listed can be assumed to be for oral consumption unless designated otherwise. In the geriatric population, intravenous (IV) antibiotics should be avoided where possible, since IV therapy often involves immobilizing the frail elderly. Dosage suggestions are in accord with accepted standards, however physicians are advised to consult the product monograph and other sources for additional information on age and condition specific dosing. This is particularly important with children, patients with renal impairment and with new or infrequently used drugs.

When prescribing for CHILDREN a general rule is not to exceed the adult daily dosage.

Prices / Costs

Wherever available, an approximate daily treatment cost has been included for most anti-infective agents. For children, a cost per kilogram per day (cost/kg/day) is estimated from available oral liquid preparations. Approximate costs were derived from the Ontario Drug Benefit (ODB) e-formulary or manufacturers' price lists. It is acknowledged that acquisition price will vary according to individual pharmacy practices, thus the estimated daily costs may not reflect all community situations. The daily cost does not include professional fees or markups. Parenteral (IV, IM) costs may vary according to jurisdiction and/or contract pricing.

Antibiotic Prescribing Pearls

Antibiotic Resistance

The incidence and adverse consequences of infections caused by antimicrobial-resistant organisms continues to increase; the spread of these organisms within the community (colonization and infection) is increased by the use of antibiotics (Conly 2002; Mulvey 2009).

Macrolide-resistant *S. pneumoniae* in Canada increased dramatically from 3.7% in 1995 to 19.0% in 2005 (Karlowsky 2009); recent data suggests it is now more than 20% (CBSN 2009). Macrolide use is the single most important driver of this and has been shown to increase the colonization of macrolide-resistant *S. pneumoniae* by 50%. The risk of resistance is greater with longer-acting than with shorter-acting macrolides (azithromycin once daily > clarithromycin BID >> erythromycin QID), thus, the risk associated with previous use of azithromycin is greater than with use of other macrolides (Karlowsky 2009; Malhotra-Kumar 2007; Vanderkooi 2005). This is also the case with macrolide resistant *S. pyogenes* (Gagliotti 2006).

Fluoroquinolone-resistance in certain regions of Canada is significant; check with your local public health for regional rates. Acquisition of a respiratory infection in a hospital or nursing home is a significant risk factor for infection with fluoroquinolone-resistant pneumococci (Adam 2009; Chen 1999; Mandell 2007; Wu 2009). Also, due to the rapid increase in quinolone resistant *N. gonorrhoeae*, quinolones are no longer preferred drugs for the empiric treatment of gonococcal infections in Canada (Ota 2009; Tapsall 2009). Ciprofloxacin resistant *E. coli* has also increased to as high as 10-15% in some areas (McGeer 2009) and should be taken into account in prescribing for urinary tract infections.

Importance of Antibiotic History in Past 3 Months

Knowledge of antimicrobial use during the three months before infection is crucial for determining appropriate therapy for a patient presenting with any infection. Review antibiotics prescribed for any type of infection in the previous three months. If there has been exposure to a particular class of antibiotics then consider selecting from an alternate class. Physicians are encouraged to limit the use of antibiotics and to avoid broad-spectrum agents with a greater propensity to select for resistant bacteria (Malhotra-Kuma 2007; Patrick 2009).

Penicillin - Cephalosporin Cross Allergy

Penicillins and cephalosporins are often the safest and most effective drugs for treating infections. Patients reporting an allergy to them are often unnecessarily prescribed inferior drugs. Current information reveals that many penicillin-allergic patients can be safely treated with certain cephalosporins. The reluctance to prescribe cephalosporin antibiotics for these patients is based on historical data that suggested the rate of cross-reactivity may be as high as 10%; a revised estimate of 0.4% cross-reactivity between penicillins (including ampicillin and amoxicillin) and first-generation cephalosporins (cefazolin, cephalexin, cefadroxil) is now suggested (Pichichero 2005). The side chains, rather than the beta-lactam ring itself, induces allergic reaction so there is no cross-reactivity between penicillins and the 2nd-generation cephalosporin cefuroxime or 3rd-generation ceftriaxone, cefotaxime, ceftazidime and cefixime (Pichichero 2005). Furthermore, a series of over 400 patients reporting a history of unspecified rash (without angioedema, bronchospasm, anaphylactic shock) on penicillin received IV cefazolin as surgical prophylaxis without any of them experiencing an allergic reaction to it (Goodman 2001).

Suggested Management of Patients who say they are Penicillin Allergic (Pennie 2010)

   a) If the "allergy" is vague and unspecified, or is a rash without angioedema, bronchospasm, anaphylactic shock, or the need for resuscitative measures, any sort of cephalosporin can be prescribed with relative safety. Such patients are at the same risk of anaphylaxis as patients reporting no history of penicillin allergy.

   b) If the "allergy" includes angioedema, bronchospasm, anaphylactic shock, or the need for resuscitative measures, then ceftriaxone, cefotaxime, ceftazidime, cefixime and cefuroxime can be given safely with no greater risk of anaphylaxis than the general population. Cefazolin, cephalexin, cefadroxil and cefprozil are best avoided, or given under controlled conditions (adrenaline at the ready) because they carry a small risk of cross-reactivity.

   c) If the patient tolerates the cephalosporin without allergic reaction, it is helpful to note the lack of reaction in the chart for the edification of future health care providers.

References: Adam 2009; Am Acad Ped 2004; Can Paed Soc 2009; CBSN 2009; Chen 1999; Conly 2002; DePestel 2008; Gagliotti 2006; Goodman 2001; Karlowsky 2009; Malhotra-Kumar 2007; Mandell 2007; McGeer 2009; Mulvey 2009; Ota 2009; Patrick 2009; Pennie 2010; Pichichero 2005; Tapsall 2009; Vanderkooi 2005; Wu 2009.

Eye Infections

Acute Conjunctivitis (Pink Eye) – Clinical Clues [1, 2, 3]

Etiology	Predisposing Factors	Signs and Symptoms
Bacterial Acute and Chronic	• **Recent contact** • **Children:** bacterial more common (~50–75%) than viral	• **Rapid onset (24h) of acute of uni/bilateral conjunctival redness** • **Gluey/sticky eyelids, especially in morning; crusts on lashes** • **Copious, thick mucopurulent discharge (white, yellow or green) at lid margin/corners, persisting throughout the day** • Eyelid redness/swelling • Discomfort or pain, possible foreign-body sensation • The more discharge, the more severe • **Mild:** very mild stickiness/erythema, no purulent discharge • **Severe:** signs of progression to periorbital cellulitis (e.g., erythema, fever, swelling) • Photophobia is a sign that the cornea is infiltrated
Gonococcal (*hyperacute*) and Chlamydial (*inclusion*) [See also pages 84 to 86]	• Emergency • Exposure to Sexually Transmitted Infection • Chlamydia and gonococcal in neonates	• **Tender pre-auricular lymphadenopathy** • **Rapid onset < 24h; rapidly progressing redness, copious discharge, lid edema** • **Usually unilateral** • Corneal perforation can occur (~10%); urgent referral • Neonatal gonococcal infection is associated with marked bilateral purulent discharge and local inflammation; chlamydial is characterized by ocular congestion, edema, and discharge that is usually more watery in nature developing a few days to several weeks after birth and lasting for 1 to 2 weeks or longer.
Viral [For herpes keratitis see page 57]	• **Recent contact** (highly contagious; viable on dry surfaces for 2 weeks or longer) • **Recent cold or flu-like symptoms ≥ 2 weeks** • **Adults:** viral is more common	• **Thin, clear, watery discharge; minimal lash crusts** • **Rapid onset uni/bilateral diffuse conjunctival redness** • **Itchy eyes and a history of conjunctivitis** • **Systemic symptoms common (e.g., sneezing, runny nose)** • Amount and character of fibrinous discharge and general ocular inflammation are used as indicators of severity • Foreign-body sensation common (burning, sandy, gritty) • Profuse tearing; eyelids red or edematous • Possible pre-auricular adenopathy; no photophobia or pain
Allergic	• **Atopic conditions** (e.g., seasonal allergies, eczema, asthma, urticaria), seasonal pollens, environmental exposure • Difficult to distinguish from viral	• **Itchy; worse with rubbing** • **Watery discharge; thin, white ropey discharge may be present** • **Bilateral diffuse conjunctival redness** • Eyelids red or edematous • Often other allergic symptoms • Use naphazoline 0.1%-pheniramine (e.g., Diopticon A) 1-2 drops QID prn. Alternatives include: olopatadine 0.1% (Patanol) 1 drop BID or ketorolac 0.5% (Ocular) 1 drop QID

1) **What is 'Pink Eye'?** Although most eye inflammations result in a pink discolouration of the eye due to dilated blood vessels, the term 'pink eye' is usually used for conjunctivitis caused by infection with a bacteria or virus. Approximately 32-50% of cases are bacterial (Rietveld 2004).

2) Most viral and bacterial conjunctivitis will resolve spontaneously; bacterial conjunctivitis has been reported to have a spontaneous remission rate of 65% by days 2 to 5 in those receiving placebo (Sheikh 2006). Conjunctival scrapings or cultures are generally not needed except in resistant or recurrent cases. The exception is *N. gonorrhoeae* infection which can progress to keratitis, corneal ulceration, endophthalmitis, scarring and blindness in a matter of hours.

3) **When may corticosteroids be indicated?** Generally, there is no role for use of steroid or antibiotic/steroid combination ophthalmic preparations in a primary care setting. Conditions where they may be helpful and where an ophthalmology consult is recommended include: corneal ulceration, keratoconjunctivitis, ocular allergy or viral keratitis.

References: AAO 2008; AAP 2012; CDC 2006; Johns Hopkins 2011; Health Canada 2000; Patel 2007; Tarabishy 2008; Rietveld 2004, 2007; Sheik 2006; Visscher 2009.

Modifying Circumstances	Probable Organism(s)	Antibiotic Choice(s)		Usual Dosage‡

Acute Conjunctivitis (Pink Eye) – Adult and Children [1, 2, 3]

Modifying Circumstances	Probable Organism(s)		Antibiotic Choice(s)	Usual Dosage‡
ADULT AND CHILDREN > 1 YEAR OF AGE	**VIRAL** Adenovirus Cosackievirus ECHO virus		**No antibiotic or antiviral indicated** (except with herpes keratitis - see page 57)	Consider cold compresses (e.g., tea bags), decongestants and/or artificial tears (AAO 2008)
	BACTERIAL [1] S. aureus S. pneumoniae H. influenzae M. catarrhalis	**OTC**	Gramicidin-polymyxin B drops (*Polysporin or Optimyxin*)	1 drop q3-4h
			Bacitracin-polymyxin B ointment (*Polysporin or Optimyxin*)	½ inch QID
		RX	Erythromycin 0.5% ointment	½-1 inch QID
			Fucidin 1% drops (Children > 2 yrs)	1 drop BID
			Sulfacetamide sodium 10% drops	1-2 drops q2-3h then taper to BID
			Trimethoprim-polymyxin B drops (*Polytrim*)	1-2 drops q3h
			Neomycin-gramicidin-polymyxin B drops (*Optimyxin PLUS*)	1-2 drops q4h
			Neomycin-bacitracin-polymyxin B ointment (*Diosporin*)	½ inch QID
			Framycetin 0.5% drops OR ointment	1-2 drops q1-2 hrs x 2-3 days if acute then reduce to BID-TID ½ inch BID-TID
			Gentamicin 0.3% drops OR ointment (Children > 6 yrs)	1-2 drops q4h then taper ½ inch q4h then BID-TID
			Tobramycin 0.3% drops OR ointment (Children > 6 yrs)	1-2 drops q4h then taper ½ inch q4h then BID-TID
PREFERRED FOR MORE SEVERE CASES (E.G., CONTACT LENSES, CORNEAL INVOLVEMENT, TREATMENT FAILURE) [2]			Besifloxacin 0.6% drops	1 drop TID x 7 days
			Ciprofloxacin 0.3% drops OR ointment	1-2 drops q2h x 2 days then q4h x 5 days ½ inch BID - TID
			Gatifloxacin 0.3% drops	1-2 drops q2h x 2 days then QID x 5 days
			Levofloxacin 0.5% drops	1-2 drops q2h x 2 days then q4h x 5 days
			Moxifloxacin 0.5% drops	1 drop TID x 7 days
			Ofloxacin 0.3% drops	1-2 drops q2-4h x 2 days then 1-2 drops QID x 5 days

Continued...

© 2013 Anti-infective Review Panel

‡ Common oral dosage ranges are provided unless otherwise stated. Consult the drug monograph for details on age and condition-specific dosing. **Page 3**

Acute Conjunctivitis (Pink Eye) – Adult and Children

1) **Bacterial conjunctivitis is usually self-limited and will often resolve spontaneously** with proper hand and eye hygiene in immune-competent individuals. While topical antibiotics are associated with significantly improved rates of early clinical remission (days 2-5), their benefit is marginal for later remission (days 6-10) (Sheikh 2005). Delayed prescribing of antibiotics is an appropriate strategy for managing acute conjunctivitis in primary care as this provides similar duration and severity of symptoms to immediate prescribing and reduces reoccurrence (Everitt 2006; Visscher 2009). Conjunctivitis in children is predominantly bacterial (*H. influenzae*).

2) **Choice of antibiotic is usually empirical with recommended duration of therapy 5 to 7 days** (AAO 2008) unless otherwise noted. Give all doses while awake. Ointment is preferred if there is excessive tearing for children and for those with poor compliance or difficulty administering.
Gentamicin and tobramycin: may damage corneal epithelium with prolonged use.
Fluoroquinolones: preferred for more serious cases, especially suspected *Pseudomonas* (e.g., contact lens wearers) or corneal involvement. Quinolones are comparable in efficacy, except for moxifloxacin, which was found to reduce symptoms and disease transmission to 2 days (Granet 2008) and to be more potent than gatifloxacin against gram-positive organisms (Kowalski 2003, 2005; Mather 2002).
Chloramphenicol (0.25% or 0.5% solution 1-2 drops q4-6h or 1% ointment) could be considered if no other option is available.

Refer if no improvement within 24-72 hours after initiating therapy or if the following develops: moderate/severe ocular pain, severe purulent discharge, diminished visual acuity, or in patients with conjunctivitis related to sexually transmitted infection.

Topical corticosteroids should be used with caution or avoided if possible, unless the patient is under the care of an ophthalmologist. Potential adverse affects include prolongation of adenoviral infections, worsening of herpes simplex virus infections or formation of corneal ulcer (AAO 2008).

3) **Counselling:**
1) Advise regarding self-limiting nature of condition
2) Both the bacterial and viral form are highly contagious for 48-72 hours; restrict contact with others 24-48 hours after treatment is initiated. Avoid sharing personal items and ensure careful handwashing
3) Cleanse affected eye(s) by wiping from the inner canthus outward using a single tissue/cotton ball
4) Clean eyelashes several times a day with weak solution of no-tears baby shampoo and warm water

References: AAO 2008; AAP 2012; AOA 2002; CAN STI 2008, 2010; Epling 2007; Everitt 2006; Granet 2008; Hovding 2008; Johns Hopkins 2011; Kowalski 2003, 2005; Mather 2002; Patel 2007; Pichichero 2011; Sheikh 2005, 2009; Silver 2005; Rhee 2007; Rietveld 2003, 2004, 2005, 2007; Tarabishy 2008; Visscher 2009; Williams 2012.

Blepharitis – Adult and Children: Clinical Clues

	Etiology	Signs and Symptoms	Management Plan
A N T E R I O R	**Seborrheic** Seborrheic dermatitis	• **Mild forms often symptom free** • Greasy, foamy scales at base of cilia margins and around lashes • Hyperemia of anterior lid margins • No ulceration/scarring • Eyelash breakage/misdirection rare • Possible burning, stinging, itching • Inflammation usually minimal	• Lid hygiene BID-TID until improved, then once daily • Patients with seborrhea of the scalp should consider using anti-seborrheic shampoos
	Bacterial *S. aureus* *S. epidermidis* *Others include:* *P. acnes,* *Corynebacteria*	• Ocular irritation/itching • Foreign body sensation • Lids sticking together • Erythema of lid margins • Scaly epidermal collarettes at base of lashes • Staining, erosion, infiltrates in lower third of cornea • Eyelash breakage/misdirection	• Lid hygiene BID-TID until improved then once daily • Tear supplements PRN • Antibiotic ointment • Corticosteroid drops or ointment if infiltrates
	Mixed Seborrhea, bacterial infection	• Inflammation of lids • Papillary and follicular hypertrophy • Conjunctival infection • Mixed lid crusting • Difficult to eradicate	• Lid hygiene BID-TID until improved then once daily • Antibiotic
P O S T E R I O R	**Meibomian gland dysfunction (MGD)** Rosacea, Seborrheic Dermatitis	• Thick lipid secretions and plugged/pouting meibomian gland orifices • Eyelid scarring with longstanding disease • Eyelash breakage unusual • No eyelid ulcerations • Chalazion (stye) - lump in the eyelid caused by inflammation of a gland • Corneal inflammation/ulceration may occur • Itching, tearing, burning sensation • Conjunctival infection	• Lid hygiene up to TID • Scalp shampoo daily • Meibomian massage/express daily • Antibiotic or antibiotic/corticosteroid ointment QHS to TID may be added when the infection has been identified clinically

Blepharitis is an inflammation of the eyelids causing red, irritated, itchy eyelids and the formation of dandruff-like scales on eyelashes. It is caused by either a bacteria or a skin condition (e.g., dandruff of the scalp or acne rosacea). It affects people of all ages. Although uncomfortable, blepharitis is not contagious and generally does not cause any permanent damage to eyesight.

Anterior blepharitis occurs at the outside front edge of the eyelid where the eyelashes are attached. **Posterior blepharitis** affects the inner edge of the eyelid that comes in contact with the eyeball.

References: AAO 2008; AOA 2003; Health Canada 2000; Jackson 2008.

Blepharitis – Adult and Children [1,2,3,4,5,6]

Modifying Circumstances	Probable Organism(s)		Antibiotic Choice(s)	Usual Dosage‡
BACTERIA OR MIXED (seborrheic/ bacterial) OR MEIBOMIAN GLAND DYSFUNCTION (MGD)	S. aureus S. epidermidis P. acnes Corynebacteria	NON-PHARMA-COLOGIC	LID HYGIENE Warm wash cloth with baby shampoo Artificial tears 4-8x/day as needed	Once Daily - BID
		FIRST LINE	Bacitracin-polymyxin ointment (Polysporin or Optimyxin)	½ inch QHS
			Erythromycin 0.5% ointment	½ inch QHS
		SECOND LINE	Gentamicin 0.3% ointment	½ inch QHS
			Tobramycin 0.3% ointment	½ inch QHS

1) **Lid hygiene is the mainstay of treatment and works best once daily or BID:** Apply hot compresses for 5 minutes to soften the scales and crusts (lid massage of the edge toward the eye with a gentle circular motion may help improve secretion), then scrub the eyelid margin and the bases of the eyelashes with a solution of water and baby shampoo (3 drops of shampoo in 90 mL water). Rinse with clear water and then remove lid debris with a dry, cotton-tipped applicator. **Tear supplements** may also be required to alleviate symptoms (AOA 2007; Rhee 2007). The patient should avoid rubbing or irritating eyelids and exposure to wind, smoke, cosmetics and other irritants. Contact lenses should not be worn during treatment.

2) **Antibiotic ointments** are helpful in the short term of an acute phase, but resistance and consequent lack of efficacy rapidly ensue if treatment is prolonged. The agents listed above may possess high rates of resistance locally in which case a fluoroquinolone (moxifloxacin or gatifloxacin) may be considered where cultures and sensitivities have not been done; use of high dose, short duration will minimize development of resistance and maximize efficacy. Ophthalmic ointments remain in contact with the lid margin for longer periods of time and are preferable to solutions; apply to lid margins and into lower conjunctival sac.

3) **Oral antibiotics:** Patients with MGD or ocular rosacea whose chronic symptoms are not responding to eyelid hygiene may benefit from oral tetracyclines (doxycycline 100 mg BID or tetracycline 250 mg QID x 2-6 weeks then taper to doxycycline 50 mg or tetracycline 250-500 mg/day). Alternatively, erythromycin 250-500 mg QID can be used. Erythromycin 30-50 mg/kg/day divided TID-QID is the drug of choice in children (Rhee 2007).

4) **Topical corticosteroids** are usually not helpful and can lead to prolongation of disease and continued colonization by bacteria. Evaluation by an ophthalmologist is generally recommended prior to initiation of topical corticosteroids. A brief course may be helpful for eyelid or ocular surface inflammation, such as in severe conjunctival infection, marginal keratitis or phlyctenules. If used, taper and discontinue once the inflammation is controlled. Long-term therapy should be avoided (AAO 2008).

5) **Antibiotic-corticosteroid combination products** have occasional applicability, but are rarely beneficial when administered without access to a careful slit lamp exam and ability to measure intraocular pressure.

6) **Refer to an ophthalmologist** if loss of visual acuity, moderate or severe pain, severe or chronic redness, corneal involvement, recurrent episodes or lack of response to therapy.

References: AAO 2008; AOA 2003; Health Canada 2000; Jackson 2008; McCulley 2000; Rhee 2007.

© 2013 Anti-infective Review Panel

Page 6   ‡ Common oral dosage ranges are provided unless otherwise stated. Consult the drug monograph for details on age and condition-specific dosing.

Respiratory Infections

Pharyngitis[1]

In general practice, approximately 80-90% of the time uncomplicated pharyngitis is NOT a Group A Streptococcal infection (i.e., Strep throat) and does not require antibiotic therapy. The following SCORECARD can assist health practitioners in the treatment (not diagnosis) of patients presenting with upper respiratory tract infection symptoms and a sore throat.

Step 1
After a clinical assessment, where you conclude the patient has an uncomplicated upper respiratory tract infection with a sore throat, determine the patient's total sore throat score by assigning points according to the following criteria:

Criteria	Points
• Temperature > 38° C	1
• Absence of Cough	1
• Swollen, tender anterior cervical nodes	1
• Tonsillar swelling or exudate	1
• Age 3-14 yr	1
• Age 15-44 yr	0
• Age ≥ 45 yr	-1

Step 2
Choose the appropriate management according to the sore throat score:

Total Score	Risk of Streptococcal Infection (%)	Suggested Management[2]
0 or less	1-2.5	• No culture or antibiotic required[2]
1	5-10	
2	11-17	• Perform culture (or office Rapid antigen test[3])
3	28-35	• Treat only if test is positive for Group A Strep.
4 or more	51-53	• Start antibiotic therapy on clinical grounds (patient has high fever or is clinically unwell and presents early in disease course). • If culture (or office Rapid antigen test[3]) is performed and result is negative then antibiotic should be discontinued.

1) Adapted from McIsaac WJ et al. JAMA 2004;291:1587-95. Score cards (i.e., McIsaac and Centor) have recently undergone a large scale validation (Fine 2012). This score should not be used in epidemic situations; in populations in which rheumatic fever remains a problem, such as First Nations communities (Madden 2009); those individuals who have a history of rheumatic fever, valvular heart disease and/or immunosuppression.

2) It is always appropriate to perform a throat culture if other clinical factors lead you to suspect Streptococcal infection (i.e., household contact with Streptococcal infection). Swab tonsils and peritonsillar pillars.

3) **If the antigen test is negative, <u>then culture is still required for children.</u> In adults, a negative antigen test alone is reasonable.**

References: Centor 2007(a,b); Fine 2012; Forward 2006; Madden 2009; Maltezou 2008; McIsaac 2004; MQIC 2008; Worrall 2007.

Modifying Circumstances	Probable Organism(s)		Antibiotic Choice(s)	Usual Dosage‡	Cost per Day

Pharyngitis – Adult [1, 2, 3]

The primary purpose of treatment is the prevention of acute rheumatic fever. Based on available evidence and, unless stated otherwise, regimens require a 10-day course in order to achieve successful treatment and prevent post-streptococcal sequelae.

ADULT	**VIRAL** 80-90% of the time, pharyngitis is not bacterial.		**No antibiotic indicated**	Viral features include: Conjunctivitis, cough, hoarseness, coryza, anterior stomatitis, discrete ulcerative lesions	
	BACTERIAL *Group A Strep* (GAS)	*FIRST LINE*	Penicillin V	300 mg (500 000 units) TID or 600 mg BID	$0.21 - $0.28
		SECOND LINE	Erythromycin	250 mg QID	$0.73
		THIRD LINE	Cephalexin	250 mg QID	$0.90
			Cefadroxil	500 mg BID	$1.68
			Cefuroxime-AX [4]	250 mg BID	$1.45
			Cefprozil [4]	250 mg BID	$0.86
			Clarithromycin	250 mg BID	$0.82
			Azithromycin	500 mg daily on first day then 250 mg daily x 4 days	$1.57

1) Approximately 20% of the population may carry *Group A Strep* asymptomatically. These individuals only need to be identified or treated if there is a family history of rheumatic fever, an outbreak of rheumatic fever, an outbreak of pharyngitis in a closed community, or repeat transmission within families (≥ 3 culture confirmed episodes of symptomatic pharyngitis). Perform swab during an asymptomatic period of patient and household members to document carrier status. Use same dosage as above .

2) Individuals who experience significant difficulties swallowing, especially if associated with drooling, presence of altered voice (so-called 'hot potato' voice) or airway obstruction (i.e., stridor) should be considered to have epiglottitis, peritonsillar abscess, or retropharyngeal abscess, until proven otherwise.

3) Recent data suggest that in adolescents and young adults (15 to 24 years), *Fusobacterium necrophorum* causes endemic pharyngitis at a rate similar to that of *Group A Strep (GAS)*. *F. necrophorum* is estimated to cause Lemierre's syndrome (a life-threatening suppurative complication) at a higher incidence than that which group A streptococcus causes acute rheumatic fever and with greater morbidity and mortality. Patients in this age group who develop bacteremic symptoms or unilateral neck swelling, should be treated empirically with penicillins or cephalosporins rather than macrolides (Centor 2009; Karkos 2009).

4) Some studies have demonstrated improved eradication rates with short-course broad-spectrum cephalosporins, however this may unnecessarily broaden the spectrum of activity of therapy and requires further investigation before being routinely recommended for use (Casey 2004; Pichichero 1997).

References: AHA 2009; Alcaide 2007; Armengol 2004; Altamimi 2009; Bisno 2004; Casey 2004, 2005(b), 2007(a); Centor 2009; Chiappini 2011; Cooper 2001; DePestal 2008; Gerber 2005; Karkos 2009; Korb 2010; IDSA 2012; Madden 2009; McIssac 2004; NICE 2008; Norrby 2003, 2004; Pichichero 2000, 2006, 2007; Quinn 2003; SIGN 2010; Snow 2001; Wessels 2011; Zhanel 2002.

© 2013 Anti-infective Review Panel

‡ Common oral dosage ranges are provided unless otherwise stated. Consult the drug monograph for details on age and condition-specific dosing.   **Page 9**

Modifying Circumstances	Probable Organism(s)	Antibiotic Choice(s)	Usual Dosage‡	Cost per Day

Pharyngitis – Children [1, 2]

The primary purpose of treatment is the prevention of acute rheumatic fever. Based on available evidence and, unless stated otherwise, regimens require a 10-day course in order to achieve successful treatment and prevent post-streptococcal sequelae.

CHILDREN				
	VIRAL 80-90% of the time, pharyngitis is not bacterial.	**No antibiotic indicated**	Viral features include: Conjunctivitis, cough, hoarseness, coryza, anterior stomatitis, discrete ulcerative lesions	
	BACTERIAL *Group A Strep (GAS)*	**FIRST LINE**	Penicillin V	≤ 27 kg: 40 mg/kg/day divided BID - TID (Maximum: 750 mg/day) > 27 kg: Use adult dose	$0.03 - $0.09/kg
			Amoxicillin	40 mg/kg/day divided BID - TID	$0.04 - $0.06/kg
		SECOND LINE	Erythromycin estolate	40 mg/kg/day (estolate) divided BID or TID	$0.06/kg
		THIRD LINE	Cephalexin	25-50 mg/kg/day divided QID	$0.05 - $0.09/kg
			Cefprozil [3]	15 mg/kg/day divided BID	$0.05/kg
			Cefuroxime-AX [3]	20 mg/kg/day divided BID	$0.14/kg
			Clarithromycin	15 mg/kg/day divided BID	$0.17/kg
			Azithromycin	12 mg/kg daily for 5 days (Maximum: 500 mg/day)	$0.24/kg

1) Approximately 20% of the population may carry Group A Strep asymptomatically. These individuals usually do not need to be identified or treated except under the following conditions: family history of rheumatic fever, outbreak of rheumatic fever, outbreak of pharyngitis in a closed community or repeat transmission within families (≥ 3 culture confirmed episodes of symptomatic pharyngitis). Perform swab during an asymptomatic period of patient and household members to document carrier status. Use same dosages as indicated.

2) Individuals who experience significant difficulties swallowing, especially if associated with drooling, presence of altered voice (so-called 'hot potato' voice) or airway obstruction (i.e., stridor) should be considered to have epiglottitis, peritonsillar abscess, or retropharyngeal abscess, until proven otherwise.

3) Some studies have demonstrated improved eradication rates with short-course broad-spectrum cephalosporins, however this may unnecessarily broaden the spectrum of activity and requires further investigation before being routinely recommended for use (Casey 2004; Pichichero 1997).

References: Am Acad Ped 2004; AHA 2009; Armengol 2004; Altamimi 2009; Bisno 2004; Brook 2006; Can Paed Soc 2009; Casey 2004, 2005(a,b), 2007(a,b); Chiappini 2011; Cohen 2004(a,b); Centor 2009; Cooper 2001; DePestal 2008; Gerber 2005; IDSA 2012; Karkos 2009; Korb 2010; McIssac 2004; NICE 2008; Norrby 2003, 2004; Pichichero 2000, 2006, 2007; Quinn 2003; Regoli 2011; SIGN 2010; Snow 2001; Wessels 2011; Zhanel 2002; Zwart 2003.

© 2013 Anti-infective Review Panel

Page 10   ‡ Common oral dosage ranges are provided unless otherwise stated. Consult the drug monograph for details on age and condition-specific dosing.

Modifying Circumstances	Probable Organism(s)		Antibiotic Choice(s)	Usual Dosage‡	Cost per Day

Epiglottitis (Supraglottitis) – Medical Emergency[1, 2, 3]

Modifying Circumstances	Probable Organism(s)		Antibiotic Choice(s)	Usual Dosage‡	Cost per Day
ADULT & CHILDREN	Adults: *Group A Strep.* *S. pneumoniae* *H. influenzae* type B (rare)	**FIRST LINE**	**Cefotaxime IV**	1 - 2 g q8h **Children:** 100 - 150 mg/kg/day divided q4-6h (Maximum: 8 g/day)	
PRIORITY IS TO ESTABLISH AIRWAY CONTROL	Children: *S. aureus* *Group A Strep.* *H. influenzae* type B (rare) *S. pneumoniae*		**Ceftriaxone IV**	1 - 2 g q24h **Children:** 75 - 100 mg/kg/day divided q12-24h (Maximum: 4 g/day)	IV costs vary according to jurisdiction and/or contract pricing.
			Cefuroxime IV	750 mg - 1.5 g q8h **Children:** 100 - 150 mg/kg/day divided q8h (Maximum: 4.5 g/day)	
		SECOND LINE	**Chloramphenicol IV**	50 - 100 mg/kg/day divided q6h **Children:** 75 - 100 mg/kg/day divided q6h (Maximum: 4 g/day)	
			Levofloxacin IV [4]	500 mg q24h	

1) Adults are also at risk of contracting this disease. This infection has almost completely disappeared in children due to immunization against *H. influenzae* type B. If epiglottitis is suspected, one should also consider bacterial tracheitis.

2) Contact an infectious disease consultant or public health regarding prophylaxis with rifampin for close contacts.

3) **Measures to secure the airway may be required.** Factors associated with a higher need for airway intervention include stridor, muffled voice, rapid clinical course and diabetes mellitus. Throat examination may precipitate airway obstruction. Corticosteroids may be used to decrease the supraglottic swelling. Humidified oxygen and racemic epinephrine may also be necessary.

4) Given the life threatening nature of this condition, levofloxacin may be considered as second line when there exists a potential serious allergy to cephalosporin. The risks from using levofloxacin (e.g., cartilage damage in children) must be balanced against the benefit of treating this life-threatening condition. Another potential alternative is TMP/SMX IV.

References: Alcaide 2007; Berger 2003; Burns 2005; Doshi 2008; Felter 2011; Hafidh 2006; Katori 2005; Kearney 2001; McEwan 2002; Sack 2002; Sick Kids 2010; Shepherd 2003; Sobol 2008; Tanner 2002.

TMP/SMX = Trimethoprim / Sulfamethoxazole   © 2013 Anti-infective Review Panel

‡ Common oral dosage ranges are provided unless otherwise stated. Consult the drug monograph for details on age and condition-specific dosing.   **Page 11**

Laryngitis [1, 2]

Viral	**No antibiotic indicated**	

1) Antibiotics are not recommended for laryngitis (Reveiz 2007).

2) Avoid smoking and throat clearing. Rest vocal chords. Symptomatic treatment: analgesics, adequate fluid intake, topical demulcents (lozenges), salt water gargles. Menthol inhalations and humidifiers may help to clear airways (NHS 2009).

References: Guppy 2005; Reveiz 2007; NHS 2009.

Croup (Laryngotracheobronchitis) [1, 2, 3]

CHILDREN	**Viral**	**No antibiotic indicated**

1) Corticosteroids have been shown to reduce the number and duration of hospitalizations, intubations and repeat visits. One dose of oral dexamethasone 0.6 mg/kg once is beneficial in the outpatient management of mild to moderate croup (Knutson 2004). This dose may be repeated in 6 to 24 hours, however there is no evidence suggesting additional benefit over a single dose.

2) In **severe** cases, epinephrine's rapid onset of action makes it beneficial because the anti-inflammatory effect of steroids may not be realized until several hours after administration. Racemic epinephrine 0.5 mL of 2.25% solution diluted in 3 mL of NS or sterile water via nebulizer is indicated in children with severe croup. The duration of effect does not exceed 2 hours and patients may be safely discharged as long as their symptoms do not recur at least 2 to 3 hours after treatment.

3) Despite a long history of use, mist therapy (e.g., "croup kettles", mist tents) have not been shown to be effective in relieving croup symptoms. Antitussive and decongestant therapy have not been studied in croup.

References: Ausejo 1999; Geelhoed 1995, 1996; Klassen 1998; Knutson 2004; Moore 2007; Rittichier 2000; Sobol 2008.

Acute Rhinitis (Colds) and Influenza (Flu) Prevention [1, 2, 3]

Viral	**No antibiotic indicated**	

1) In previously healthy individuals, the diagnosis of nonspecific upper respiratory tract infection should be used to denote an acute infection in which sinus, pharyngeal and lower airway symptoms, although frequently present, are not prominent. If symptoms are severe, and especially when accompanied by muscle aches and fatigue, then consider influenza and parainfluenza infections (Gonzales 2001).

2) Purulent secretions (thick, opaque or discoloured) from the nares or throat are common and do not predict bacterial infection. Antibiotics are not recommended in previously healthy individuals and do not enhance disease resolution (Arroll 2005; NICE 2008; Rosenstein 1998; Spurling 2007).

3) Counsel patients to drink plenty of fluids. Saline (nasal drops/sprays/rinses/gargles), analgesics and decongestants (Latte 2007; Taverner 2007) may be recommended to provide short-term symptomatic relief. Cough and cold medications are NOT recommended in the pediatric population (Basco 2009; Health Canada 2008; Taverner 2007). Evidence suggests that North American ginseng extract (CVT-E002 = COLD-FX), vitamin C, echinacea, or zinc may be of benefit in reducing the frequency, duration and severity of colds. Studies have shown that North American ginseng extract can prevent influenza symptoms in healthy adults, nursing home seniors and in those taking the influenza vaccine.

References: Arroll 2005; Barrett 2002; Basco 2009; Caruso 2007; Douglas 2004; Fahey 1998; Goel 2010; Gonzales 2001; Health Canada 2008; Hemilä 2007; Jensen 2008; Latte 2007; Linde 2006; Marshall 2004; McElhaney 2004, 2006; Melchart 2004; NICE 2008; Predy 2005; Rosenstein 1998; Snow 2001; Spurling 2007; Taverner 2007; Timmer 2008; Wu 2007.

© 2013 Anti-infective Review Panel

Page 12   ‡ Common oral dosage ranges are provided unless otherwise stated. Consult the drug monograph for details on age and condition-specific dosing.

Modifying Circumstances	Probable Organism(s)	Antibiotic Choice(s)	Usual Dosage‡	Cost per Day

Seasonal Influenza – *Post-exposure Antiviral Prophylaxis* [1, 2]

This chart pertains to seasonal influenza only; for latest updates on prevention and treatment of the pandemic H1N1 strain, please contact your local or provincial Medical Officer of Health or consult: www.phac-aspc.gc.ca

Vaccination and regular hand washing are the primary prevention strategies. Antiviral agents should not be used for post-exposure chemoprophylaxis in healthy children or adults. Prudent use of anti-viral medications is advised to minimize development of resistance to these agents. See below for when to consider chemoprophylaxis. [3]

Note: Begin prophylaxis within 36h after exposure if using zanamivir; within 48h for other agents.				
1-12 years old	Influenza A or B	**Oseltamivir** [1, 2, 5]	Consult product monograph	75 mg: $3.90
> 12 years old	Influenza A or B	**Oseltamivir** [1, 2, 5]	75 mg once daily x 10 days	$3.90
≥ 7 years old	Influenza A or B	**Zanamivir** [2, 4]	10 mg (2 inhalations x 5 mg) once daily x 10 days	10 mg: $3.70

Amantadine

Due to issues of resistance, amantadine is not currently recommended for the treatment or prophylaxis of influenza A or B (AAMI 2012/2013; CDC 2011; PHAC 2012).

1) **Note circulating strain and possible resistance patterns prior to initiating therapy.**

2) **Pregnancy/Lactation:** limited data suggest oseltamivir is not a human teratogen; due to more data, it is preferred over zanamivir during pregnancy. Both agents are compatible with breastfeeding (Tanaka 2009).
   Pediatric: Limited evidence exists for the efficacy of anti-virals for prophylaxis in children (Allen 2006; Galvao 2008); while experience with their use is increasing, there is very little data in infants and young children (Can Paed Soc 2012).

3) **Consider chemoprophylaxis in:**

   • Persons who are at higher risk for complications of influenza and are a close contact of a person with confirmed, probable, or suspected seasonal influenza during that person's infectious period.

   • Health care and public health workers, or first responders who have had a recognized, unprotected close contact exposure to a person with confirmed, probable, or suspected influenza during infectious period.

   • Institutional (LTC and hospital) settings: Prophylaxis begins when at least two residents develop acute flu-like illness within 72h of each other and have laboratory-proven illness. Prophylaxis is recommended for a minimum of 2 weeks and up to 1 week after the last known case is identified.

   • Household settings: Prophylaxis may be considered in unaffected vulnerable family members upon diagnosis of an index case and continued for 10 days. Consideration may be given to extending duration of prophylaxis up to 14 days if the index case is a child or elderly individual as they may continue to shed virus for up to 14 days after onset.

   • Within 5 days of a community outbreak prophylaxis with zanamivir 10 mg once daily for 28 days may be considered (Can Paed Soc 2012; PHAC 2012).

4) Some patients have had bronchospasm (wheezing) or serious breathing problems when using zanamivir. Many, but not all, of these patients had asthma or COPD. Due to the risk of side effects and questionable efficacy, it is not recommended for use in these patients. Asthma or COPD patients are advised to have a fast-acting inhaled bronchodilator available if zanamivir is to be used (CPS 2012).

5) For dosing of oseltamivir in renal impairment, consult oseltamivir (Tamiflu) product monograph (CPS 2012) and AMMI 2012/2013 guidelines (www.ammi.ca).

References: AAMI 2012/2013; AAP 2012; Allen 2006; Alves 2008; Aoki 2012; Can Paed Soc 2012, 2013; CCDR 2008; CDC 2011; CID 2007; Cooper 2003; CPS 2012; Deonandan 2007; Fiore 2008; Galvao 2008; Hayden 2004; Harper 2009; Jefferson 2004, 2006, 2008, 2009, 2010; Kiso 2004; Matheson 2007; NACI 2013; NICE 2008; PHAC 2012; PHO 2012; Shun-Shin 2009; Tanaka 2009; Welliver 2001; WHO 2010.

© 2013 Anti-infective Review Panel

‡ Common oral dosage ranges are provided unless otherwise stated. Consult the drug monograph for details on age and condition-specific dosing. **Page 13**

Modifying Circumstances	Probable Organism(s)	Antibiotic Choice(s)	Usual Dosage‡	Cost per Day

Seasonal Influenza – Treatment for those at Risk [1, 2]

This chart pertains to seasonal influenza only; for latest updates on prevention and treatment of the pandemic H1N1 strain, please contact your local or provincial Medical Officer of Health or consult: www.phac-aspc.gc.ca

In most healthy individuals the flu is self-limiting; treatment includes rest, fluid intake and non-prescription analgesics. Anti-viral medications are not a substitute for influenza vaccination; they should be considered when influenza is known to be circulating and the individual is at risk of developing complications. Note existing strains and possible resistance patterns prior to initiating therapy. Prudent use of anti-viral medications is advised to minimize development of resistance (Hurt 2010).

Begin antiviral treatment within 36-48 hours of onset of symptoms; effect is negligible after this time. The 48 hour window may be extended if significant immunodeficiency or progressive respiratory disease (CDC 2010; Allen 2006).

1-12 years old	Influenza A or B	**Oseltamivir** [2, 3]	Consult product monograph	75 mg: $3.90
> 12 years old	Influenza A or B	**Oseltamivir** [2, 3]	75 mg BID for 5 days	$7.80
≥ 7 years old	Influenza A or B	**Zanamivir** [2, 4]	10 mg (2 inhalations x 5 mg) BID for 5 days	$7.39

Amantidine:

Due to issues of resistance, amantadine is not currently recommended for the treatment or prophylaxis of influenza A or B (AAMI 2012/2013; CDC 2011; PHAC 2012).

1) When influenza is known to be circulating in the community, suspect patient has influenza if some or all of the following are present: fever/chills, abrupt onset of constitutional and respiratory signs and symptoms, myalgia, headache, severe malaise, loss of appetite and non-productive cough.

2) Treatment with anti-virals in healthy adults is not considered cost-effective since benefits in terms of clinical response are limited and treatment must be started immediately. They should be reserved for more complicated moderate-severe presentations and those with **risk factors, including** those with underlying comorbidities (chronic pulmonary disease, chronic kidney disease, immunocompromised, hemoglobinopathies, metabolic disease) and persons living in closed or semi-closed institutionalized settings.

   Pediatric: Overall benefit of anti-virals in otherwise healthy pediatric patients is negligible (Witley 2001); time to resolution of symptoms and/or return to normal activities, by 0.5-1.5 days, were significant in only two trials; they have little effect on asthma exacerbations or the use of antibiotics (Shun-Shin 2009). There is limited evidence of specific benefit in children 'at risk'; Piedra (2009) reported that use of oseltamivir in children with a chronic medical condition decreased respiratory illness, otitis media and hospitalizations. Antiviral therapy should be considered if the illness is severe enough to require hospitalization, the illness is progressive, severe or complicated, regardless of previous health status, or the patient is at high risk for severe disease. Parents of children for whom antiviral therapy is not recommended should be advised of symptoms and signs of worsening illness that might warrant reassessment. While experience with the use of antivirals in children is increasing, there is very little data in infants and young children (Can Paed Soc 2012). Although oseltamivir is not approved in Canada for treatment of seasonal influenza in infants under one year, it was temporarily approved for this use on the basis of a favourable risk-to-benefit ratio during the 2009 H1N1 pandemic. Oseltamivir use for 2012/2013 seasonal influenza in children younger than one year of age should be handled on a case-by-case basis based on severity of illness (Aoki 2012; Can Paed Soc 2012).

3) For dosing of oseltamivir in renal impairment, consult oseltamivir (Tamiflu) product monograph (CPS 2012) and AMMI 2012/2013 guidelines (www.ammi.ca).

4) Some patients have had bronchospasm (wheezing) or serious breathing problems when using zanamivir. Many, but not all, of these patients had asthma or COPD. Due to the risk of side effects, it is not recommended for use in these patients. If zanamivir is used in asthma or COPD patients, they should have a fast-acting inhaled bronchodilator available (CPS 2012).

References: Allen 2006; Alves 2008; AAP 2012; AMMI 2012/2013; Aoki 2012; Can Paed Soc 2012, 2013; CDC 2011; CDI 2007; Cooper 2003; CPS 2012; Fiore 2011; Galvao 2008; Harper 2009; Hurt 2010; Jefferson 2006, 2010; Kiso 2004; MacDonald 2010; Matheson 2007; NICE 2008; PHAC 2012; Piedra 2009; Tanaka 2009; Shun-Shin 2009; Whitley 2001; WHO 2010.

© 2013 Anti-infective Review Panel

Page 14   ‡ Common oral dosage ranges are provided unless otherwise stated. Consult the drug monograph for details on age and condition-specific dosing.

Modifying Circumstances	Probable Organism(s)	Antibiotic Choice(s)		Usual Dosage‡	Cost per Day

Otitis Externa (Swimmer's Ear) – Adult & Children: Acute [1,2]

Modifying Circumstances	Probable Organism(s)	Antibiotic Choice(s)		Usual Dosage‡	Cost per Day
WITHOUT TYMPANIC MEMBRANE PERFORATION	P. aeruginosa Coliforms S. aureus	FIRST LINE	BURO-SOL[3] otic solution	2-3 drops TID or QID	15 mL bottle: $4.05
		SECOND LINE	CORTISPORIN[2,4] otic solution	4 drops TID or QID **Children:** 3 drops TID or QID	10 mL: $13.10
			SOFRACORT[2,5] otic solution	2-3 drops TID or QID	8 mL: $14.96
			GARASONE[2,6] otic solution	3-4 drops TID	7.5 mL: $9.61
			CIPRODEX[7] otic suspension	4 drops BID	7.5 mL: $27.08
TYMPANIC MEMBRANE DEFECT			CIPRODEX[7] otic suspension	4 drops BID	7.5 mL: $27.08

1) Cultures not routinely indicated. Pulling on the pinna may be extremely painful in otitis externa, but is usually tolerated in patients with otitis media (Rosenfeld 2006). This may be helpful in differentiating otitis externa from otitis media, unless both conditions exist.
   PROPHYLAXIS: After swimming, attempt to remove as much moisture from external auditory canal as possible. A few inexpensive approaches have been suggested, such as warm air from a hair dryer, tilting the head to allow draining and/or in the **PRESENCE OF AN INTACT TYMPANIC MEMBRANE** adding a few drops of vinegar to the ear (with or without equal amounts of either water or isopropyl alcohol). Avoid use of cotton-tipped swabs or objects, such as bobby pins to clean ears; this can cause further excoriation of the canal skin.
   TREATMENT: Aural toilet is important if there is significant debris in the ear that can be easily reached. If ear is severely swollen, use of a merocel wick is recommended. Management should include an assessment of pain. If a defect of the tympanic membrane cannot be ruled out, based on history or physical examination, then management should proceed as if there is a defect.
   INFECTION ONLY: A steroid is useful where there is an underlying dermatitis. If it appears to be purely an infection, a product without a steroid can be used (e.g., polysporin or polysporin/lidocaine 1-2 drops QID). If it persists after 7 days, then reassess, consider referral. Prolonged use of combination steroid/antibiotic may result in secondary fungal infection and development of mycelial plug. Oral antimicrobial therapy is usually not considered unless condition extended beyond the ear canal or host factors indicate a need for systemic therapy. Factors that will modify management include: nonintact tympanic membrane, tympanostomy tube, diabetes, immunocompromised state, prior radiation therapy (Rosenfeld 2006).
2) **OTOTOXICITY: Health Canada advises that gentamicin containing ear drops SHOULD NOT BE USED in patients with non-intact eardrum (broken, perforated or absent eardrum or with presence of surgical ear tubes). In general, patients should be advised to stop treatment immediately if hearing loss, tinnitus, vertigo or imbalance is noted. Refer to specialist if condition does not settle (Bath 1999; Hannley 2000; Health Canada 2002; Matz 2004; Roland 2004(c)). Since this is a class effect, caution should also be used with other aminoglycosides (e.g., CORTISPORIN, SOFRACORT) containing drops - for suggested treatment see footnote 7.**
3) BURO-SOL contains 0.5% aluminum acetate and 0.03% benzethonium chloride in dilute acetic acid solution. This is considered as initial treatment instead of topical antibiotics because of its lower toxicity, avoids resistance, and is less expensive (Clayton 1990).
4) CORTISPORIN contains 10000 U polymyxin, 5 mg neomycin and 10 mg hydrocortisone per mL.
5) SOFRACORT contains 5 mg framycetin, 0.05 mg of gramicidin and 0.5 mg dexamethasone per mL.
6) GARASONE contains 3 mg of gentamicin and 1 mg of betamethasone per mL.
7) CIPRODEX contains 3 mg of ciprofloxacin and 1 mg of dexamethsone per mL. Should be considered treatment of choice in presence of tympanic membrane defect or if integrity of tympanic membrane cannot be verified.

References: Am Acad Peds 2006; Bath 1999; Clayton 1990; Drehobl 2008; Hannley 2000; Health Canada 2002; Hui 2013 (Can Paed Soc); Kaushik 2010; Matz 2004; Mösges 2007; Osguthorpe 2006; Pappas 2008; Rahman 2007; Roland 2004(c), 2008; Rosenfeld 2006 (a, b); Schwartz 2006; Van Balen 2003; Wall 2009; Weber 2004.

Modifying Circumstances	Probable Organism(s)		Antibiotic Choice(s)	Usual Dosage‡	Cost per Day

Otitis Externa – Adult: Necrotizing (Malignant) [1, 2, 3, 4]

Modifying Circumstances	Probable Organism(s)		Antibiotic Choice(s)	Usual Dosage‡	Cost per Day
	P. aeruginosa	ORAL THERAPY	Ciprofloxacin [4]	750 mg BID	$2.56
		IV THERAPY	Ciprofloxacin IV alone	400 mg q12h	
			Ticarcillin/Clavulanate IV	3.1 g q4-6h	
			Piperacillin/Tazobactam IV	3 g/0.375 g q6h	
			Piperacillin IV	3 - 4 g q4-6h	
			Imipenem/Cilastatin IV	500 mg q6h	IV costs vary according to jurisdiction and/or contract pricing.
			Meropenem IV	1 g q8h	
			Ceftazidime IV	1 - 2 g q8h	
			± ONE of the following:		
			Gentamicin IV [5] OR	4 - 7 mg/kg q24h	
			Tobramycin IV [5] OR	4 - 7 mg/kg q24h	
			Amikacin IV [5]	15 - 20 mg/kg q24h	

1) Necrotizing otitis externa is defined as an invasive infection of the external auditory canal and includes bone involvement. Necrotizing otitis externa is extremely rare in childhood, unless there is an underlying immunosuppressive disorder present (e.g., leukemia, Di George's Syndrome, etc.). Admission to hospital for IV therapy is recommended until stabilized then switch to oral therapy following culture. Refer to a specialist.

2) Includes the elderly and individuals with diabetes mellitus and/or who are immunocompromised.

3) Treat from 4 to 8 weeks; local treatment with topical antibiotic drops usually required concomitantly.

4) When clinical condition allows, consider oral ciprofloxacin. If parenteral therapy is required, the single agents listed above generally have excellent coverage for *pseudomonas*. Initiate treatment with double coverage if uncertainty regarding pathogen; once patient stabilizes discontinue the aminoglycoside.

5) For more information on aminoglycoside dosing, see page 109.

References: Handzel 2003; Levenson 1991; Rosenfeld 2006; Van Balen 2003.

Otitis Externa – Otomycosis [1, 2]

Modifying Circumstances	Probable Organism(s)		Antibiotic Choice(s)	Usual Dosage‡	Cost per Day
ADULT & CHILDREN	FUNGAL Candida albicans Aspergillus niger	FIRST LINE	Clotrimazole 1 % cream	Apply BID (AM and HS)	30 g: $6.64
			Tolnaftate 1 % cream	Apply BID (AM and HS)	50 g: $9.50
			LOCACORTEN VIOFORM drops [3]	2-3 drops BID	10 mL: $15.16

1) Consider referral to a specialist. Rule out diabetes if recurrent. Predisposing factors include: absence of cerumen, high humidity or temperature, aquatic sports, local trauma, prolonged use of topical antibiotic.

2) If no response is seen with clotrimazole or tolnaftate cream (1 to 3 weeks duration), consider *Aspergillus niger* as a possible cause and treat with an agent that will cover (i.e., ketoconazole, itraconazole).

3) LOCACORTEN-VIOFORM: Each 10 mL contains flumethasone pivalate 0.02% and clioquinol 1%.

References: Garry 2007; Gutiérrez 2005; Ho 2006; Jackman 2005; Munguia 2007; Osguthorpe 2006.

Modifying Circumstances	Probable Organism(s)	Antibiotic Choice(s)	Usual Dosage‡	Cost per Day

Otitis Media – Adult: Acute

Modifying Circumstances	Probable Organism(s)	Antibiotic Choice(s)	Usual Dosage‡	Cost per Day
WITHOUT TYMPANIC MEMBRANE PERFORATION	*S. pneumoniae* **FIRST** *H. influenzae* **LINE** *M. catarrhalis* **SECOND** *Group A Strep.* **LINE** *S. aureus*	**Amoxicillin**	500 mg TID	$1.03
		Amoxicillin/Clavulanate	500 mg TID or 875 mg BID	$2.00
		Cefprozil	250-500 mg BID	$0.86 - $1.70
		Cefuroxime-AX	250-500 mg BID	$1.45 - $2.87
		Clarithromycin	250-500 mg BID	$0.82 - $1.65
		Azithromycin	500 mg daily on first day then 250 mg daily x 4 days	$1.57
		TMP/SMX [1]	2 tabs BID or 1 DS tab BID	$0.08 - $0.24
CHRONIC TYMPANIC MEMBRANE PERFORATION OR VENTILATION TUBES [2]	*S. aureus* *P. aeruginosa* *Viridans Streptococcus species*	**CIPRODEX** [3] **otic suspension**	4 drops BID	7.5 mL: $27.08

1) Increased pneumococcal and *H. influenzae* resistance rates make TMP/SMX a less desirable agent.
2) A topical fluoroquinolone/dexamethasone preparation is suggested for uncomplicated acute otitis media in the presence of a chronic tympanic membrane perforation or ventilation tubes. The clinical presentation is that of a painless discharge. Adjunctive systemic antibiotic therapy may be required if there is evidence of systemic illness, where there has been spread of infection beyond the middle and external ear, in treatment failures or special populations (e.g., immunocompromised states) (Roland 2003, 2004(a, c)).
3) CIPRODEX contains 3 mg of ciprofloxacin and 1 mg of dexamethsone per mL.

References: Hendley 2002; Roland 2003, 2004(a, c).

Antibiotics and Acute Otitis Media

A Guide to *Watchful Waiting* for 48 to 72 hours:

The high spontaneous recovery rate (80% to 90%) of acute otitis media may warrant watchful waiting for 48-72 hours before starting antibiotic therapy in previously healthy children (Can Paed Soc 2009). Most children do very well with this approach and are thereby spared the risks associated with repeated antibiotic prescriptions. Similar outcomes with placebo and antibiotics have been documented (84% vs 93%) (Le Saux 2005). Conditional 'wait and see' prescriptions have been proven useful in treating acute otitis media (Spiro 2006).

Children greater than age 2 years:

Give acetaminophen, ibuprofen or other analgesic for 2 or 3 days to treat the earache. There is insufficient evidence to know whether analgesic ear drops are effective or not (Foxlee 2006). Advise parents to seek immediate medical reassessment if:
- Symptoms worsen
- New symptoms appear (e.g., rash, drowsiness, difficulty breathing, vomiting)

If symptoms do not improve after 2-3 days (fever, ear pain, fussiness):
- Verify diagnosis of acute otitis media
- Start antibiotic therapy
- See next page for suggested antibiotic choices and doses
- Duration of antibiotic therapy 5 days (works as well as 10 days at this age)

Children 6 months to 2 years:

Watchful waiting is only appropriate if the parents can observe their child for 48-72 hours with assurance of appropriate medical follow-up.
Give acetaminophen, ibuprofen or other analgesic for 2 or 3 days to treat the earache.
Advise parents to seek immediate medical reassessment if:
- Symptoms worsen
- New symptoms appear (e.g., rash, drowsiness, difficulty breathing, vomiting)

Reassess the child at 24 hours to look for signs of more serious illness that may be confused with acute otitis media.
If symptoms do not improve after 2-3 days (fever, ear pain, fussiness):
- Verify diagnosis of acute otitis media
- Start antibiotic therapy
- See next page for suggested antibiotic choices and doses
- Duration of antibiotic therapy 10 days

Children under age 6 months:

Acute otitis media is a difficult diagnosis to make in this age group. Establishing an accurate diagnosis is particularly important at this vulnerable age.

Watchful waiting is not recommended if acute otitis media is reasonably certain; on the other hand, giving antibiotics for uncertain indications is not appropriate and may be dangerous. Duration of therapy is 10 days.

References: Am Acad Peds 2006; Can Paed Soc 2009; Christian-Koop 2010; Coco 2010; Damoiseaux 2000; Del Mar 1997; Foxlee 2006; Froom 1997; Glasziou 2003; Hoberman 2011; Le Saux 2005; McCormick 2005; Pichichero 2008; Piglansky 2003; Rosenfeld 1994; Spiro 2006; Tan 2008; Vernacchio 2007.

Modifying Circumstances	Probable Organism(s)	Antibiotic Choice(s)		Usual Dosage‡	Cost per Day

Otitis Media – Children: Acute [1, 2, 3, 4]

Modifying Circumstances	Probable Organism(s)	Antibiotic Choice(s)		Usual Dosage‡	Cost per Day
WITHOUT TYMPANIC MEMBRANE PERFORATION	S. pneumoniae H. influenzae M. catarrhalis	FIRST LINE	Amoxicillin [5]	80 mg/kg/day divided BID or TID (Maximum: 3 grams/day)	$0.05/kg
		SECOND LINE	Amoxicillin/Clavulanate [5, 6]	40-80 mg/kg/day amoxicillin divided BID (Maximum daily dose - see amoxicillin above)	$0.07 - $0.14/kg
			Cefprozil	30 mg/kg/day divided BID	$0.07/kg
		THIRD LINE	Cefuroxime-AX	30-40 mg/kg/day divided BID	$0.19 - $0.26/kg
			Clarithromycin [7]	15 mg/kg/day divided BID	$0.17/kg
			Azithromycin [7]	10 mg/kg/day on first day then 5 mg/kg/day x 4 days or 10 mg/kg/day once daily x 3 days	$0.18/kg $0.20/kg
			TMP/SMX [8]	5-10 mg/kg/day trimethoprim divided BID	$0.02 - $0.03/kg
CHRONIC TYMPANIC MEMBRANE PERFORATION OR VENTILATION TUBES [9]	S. aureus P. aeruginosa Viridans Streptococcus species		CIPRODEX [10] otic suspension	4 drops BID x 5 days	7.5 mL: $27.08

Continued ...

TMP/SMX = Trimethoprim / Sulfamethoxazole   © 2013 Anti-infective Review Panel

‡ Common oral dosage ranges are provided unless otherwise stated. Consult the drug monograph for details on age and condition-specific dosing.   **Page 19**

Otitis Media - Children: Acute

1) Antibiotics are more likely a consideration in infants < 6 months old and in severe illness that consists of presence of moderate to severe ear pain with fever ≥ 39°C, bilateral acute otitis media, systemic features, such as vomiting or severe local signs (e.g., perforation with purulent discharge) (AAP 2004; Rovers 2006).

2) **Otitis Media with Effusion (OME)** is the presence of fluid in the middle ear without signs or symptoms of acute ear infection and should be distinguished from acute otitis media (acute onset, purulent middle ear effusion and inflammation). OME may occur spontaneously because of poor eustachian tube function or as an inflammatory response following acute otitis media. Although bacteria have been eradicated, middle ear effusion may persist for up to 1 month in 50% of patients and up to 3 months in 10% of patients. If middle ear fluid is detected in asymptomatic children during follow-up visits, it is not necessary to continue antibiotic therapy or switch to a second line agent (Dowell 1998). Seventy-five percent to 90% of residual OME after an acute otitis media episode resolves spontaneously by 3 months. Avoiding exposure to passive smoking is the single most effective modifiable factor in preventing OME in children. Antihistamines and/or decongestants do not help and may cause harm (Griffin 2006). Long-term benefits of antibiotic therapy with or without oral steroids has not been demonstrated (AAP 2004).

3) **Prophylaxis of Recurrent Otitis Media:** Breast feed at least 6 months if possible, avoid supine bottle feeding, reduce and eliminate pacifier use in second 6 months and eliminate second hand smoke. Antibiotic prophylaxis is generally not recommended in the management of recurrent otitis media. The minimal benefit (decreasing recurrences by approximately one episode per year) is felt to be outweighed by the high risk of developing antibiotic resistance during the prolonged use of antibiotics. In high risk children, those who have experienced 3 episodes of acute otitis media in the previous 6 months or 4 episodes in the previous 12 months, a larger absolute benefit may be likely since antibiotics given once or twice daily will reduce the number of episodes of acute otitis media per year from around 3 to around 1.5 (Leach 2006).

4) **Duration of therapy:** 5 days for children older than 2 years of age with uncomplicated otitis media (Kozyrskyj 1998); 10 days for younger children or children of any age with complications (e.g., perforated eardrum or recurrent acute otitis media).

5) Higher doses have been recommended to adequately eradicate resistant *S. pneumoniae* (Am Acad Peds 2004; Can Paed Soc 2009). A standard 40 mg/kg/day dose could be considered, but not necessarily preferred, in children older than 2 years without risk factors including recent antibiotic use, use of daycare, recent episode of acute otitis media, treatment failure or early recurrence, or who live in communities where resistance has been a recognized problem. 80 mg/kg/day is recommended for children 2 years and younger and/or in daycare and/or who have had antibiotics in the past 3 months. Maximum dose of amoxicillin is 3 g daily (Christian-Kopp 2010).

6) The BID preparation has a lowered clavulanic acid content to improve its tolerance. If less clavulanic acid content is preferred, consider using a combination of amoxicillin 40 mg/kg/day plus amoxicillin/clavulanate 40 mg/kg/day (amoxicillin component) both divided BID (Can Paed Soc 2009).

7) Not appropriate for children ≤ 3 years of age with high fever who may have bacteremia. Pneumo-coccal meningitis has been reported to develop in young children while taking these medications.

8) Increased pneumococcal and *H. influenzae* resistance rates make TMP/SMX a less desirable agent.

9) **Uncomplicated acute otitis media in the presence of a chronic TM perforation or ventilation tubes:** Clinical presentation is that of a painless discharge; a topical fluoroquinolone/dexamethasone preparation is suggested for 5 days. Topical ciprofloxacin/dexamethasone was found to be superior to oral AM/CL in the median time to cessation of otorrhea (4 days vs 7 days), clinical cure rates (85% vs 59%) and adverse effects profile (Dohar 2006). Adjunctive systemic antibiotic therapy may be required if there is evidence of systemic illness; where there has been spread of infection beyond the middle and external ear; in treatment failures or special populations (e.g., immunocompromised) (Roland 2003, 2004 (a, b)).

10) CIPRODEX contains 3 mg of ciprofloxacin and 1 mg of dexamethsone per mL.

References: Am Acad Peds 2004, 2006; Can Paed Soc 2009; Christian-Kopp 2010; Dohar 2006; Dowell 1998, 1999; Garbutt 2004; Griffin 2006; Hendley 2002; Kelley 2000; Kozyrskyj 1998; Le Saux 2005; Leach 2006; McCormick 2005; Piglansky 2003; Pichichero 2008; Roland 2003, 2004 (a, b); Rovers 2006, 2007; Schrag 2001; SIGN 2003; Van Kerkhoven 2003; Vernacchio 2007.

Otitis Media – Chronic Suppurative: Adult & Children [1, 2, 3, 4]

Modifying Circumstances	Probable Organism(s)	Antibiotic Choice(s)		Usual Dosage[‡]	Cost per Day
SAFE (Due to mucosal disease)	S. aureus S. pneumoniae Proteus sp. Klebsiella sp. E. coli P. aeruginosa	**FIRST LINE**	**CIPRODEX**[5]	4 drops BID	7.5 mL: $27.08
		SECOND LINE	**CORTISPORIN**[4, 6]	3-4 drops TID or QID	10 mL: $13.10
			SOFRACORT[4, 7]	2-3 drops TID or QID	8 mL: $14.96
			GARASONE[4, 8]	3-4 drops TID	7.5 mL: $9.61
		Oral Antibiotics	See comment #1		
DANGEROUS (Due to the ingrowth of stratified squamous epithelium into the middle ear) Typically requires a surgical consult. Antibiotics useful in the interim.	P. aeruginosa E. coli Klebsiella sp. Proteus sp. S. pneumoniae S. aureus	**FIRST LINE**	**CIPRODEX**[5]	4 drops BID	7.5 mL: $27.08
		SECOND LINE	**CORTISPORIN**[4, 6]	3-4 drops TID or QID	10 mL: $13.10
			SOFRACORT[4, 7]	2-3 drops TID or QID	8 mL: $14.96
			GARASONE[4, 8]	3-4 drops TID	7.5 mL: $9.61
		Oral Antibiotics	**ONE of the above topical agents + ONE of the following** (see comment #1):		
			Ciprofloxacin	500-750 mg BID **Children:** 20-30 mg/kg/day divided BID	$1.40 - $2.56
			Levofloxacin	500 mg once daily **Children:** Limited experience	$1.37
			Moxifloxacin	400 mg once daily **Children:** Limited experience	$6.03

Continued ...

© 2013 Anti-infective Review Panel

‡ Common oral dosage ranges are provided unless otherwise stated. Consult the drug monograph for details on age and condition-specific dosing.

Otitis Media - Chronic Suppurative

1) By definition, **chronic suppurative otitis media (CSOM)** is a term used to describe either a recurrent or a persistent bacterial infection of the middle ear cleft (Paradise 2005). Hallmark features include the presence of a tympanic membrane perforation, a conductive hearing loss of varying degrees and the presence of malodorous aural discharge.

   - Clinically chronic suppurative otitis media is divided into either "SAFE" (due to chronic mucosal disease) or "DANGEROUS" due to the ingrowth of stratified squamous epithelium into the middle ear (cholesteatoma).

   - With regards to "SAFE" CSOM and a typically **dry** ear, any acute infection is likely due to common organisms that cause acute otitis media. Hence, it can be appropriate to prescribe only an oral antibiotic (those used to treat acute otitis media; cephalexin would also be acceptable), however specific otic drops (i.e., fluoroquinolone plus steroids) are equally effective and less likely to produce systemic side effects.

   - In those individuals with a **chronic discharging (wet) ear,** regardless of whether it is the so called "safe" or "dangerous" type, the organisms tend to be polymicrobial (usually gram-negatives and especially pseudomonas aeruginosa). Initial treatment generally requires a combination of appropriate topical and oral fluoroquinolones. Aminoglycoside containing drops should be used with caution as they can be ototoxic in the presence of a TM perforation. Referral to a specialist under the circumstances is generally recommended as recurrent infections are not unusual.

2) Referral to ENT specialist is recommended in the following situations:

   - Those individuals with a history of CSOM who experience acute pain, facial paralysis, vertigo and other complications
   - Those individuals with cholesteatoma
   - Those individuals with recalcitrant CSOM

3) Treatment with antibiotics alone (topical or oral) is rarely successful unless there is careful cleaning of the external canal and frequent microdebridements as often as necessary to keep canal clean and dry.

4) **OTOTOXICITY: In the presence of a TYMPANIC MEMBRANE DEFECT, the risk of ototoxicity (primarily vestibular) with topical aminoglycosides increases with duration of therapy, particularly beyond seven days or when the medication is placed into dry middle ear spaces. Health Canada advises that gentamicin containing ear drops SHOULD NOT BE USED in patients with non-intact eardrum (broken, perforated or absent eardrum or with presence of surgical ear tubes). As this is a class effect, caution should also be used with other aminoglycosides (e.g., CORTISPORIN, SOFRACORT) containing drops. In general, patients should be advised to stop treatment immediately if hearing loss, tinnitus, vertigo or imbalance is noted. Refer to specialist if condition does not settle (Bath 1999; Hannley 2000; Health Canada 2002; Matz 2004; Roland 2004 (c)).**

5) CIPRODEX: 3 mg of ciprofloxacin, 1 mg of dexamethsone per mL.

6) CORTISPORIN: 10000 U polymyxin, 5 mg neomycin, 10 mg hydrocortisone per mL.

7) SOFRACORT: 5 mg framycetin, 0.05 mg of gramicidin, 0.5 mg dexamethasone per mL.

8) GARASONE: 3 mg of gentamicin, 1 mg of betamethasone per mL.

References: Am Acad Peds 2004, 2006; Acuin 2004; Bath 1999; Dohar 1998; Hannley 2000; Health Canada 2002; Leach 2006; Matz 2004; Pappas 2006; Paradise 2005; Roland 2004 (c); Weber 2004.

Modifying Circumstances	Probable Organism(s)	Antibiotic Choice(s)	Usual Dosage[‡]	Cost per Day

Sinusitis – Adult: Acute [1, 2, 3]

Only a small percentage (less than 2%) of viral upper respiratory infections are complicated by bacterial sinusitis (Hickner 2001). Most cases of acute sinusitis are viral and resolve within 5 to 7 days without the need for antibiotics (Ahouvuo-Saloranta 2010; Williamson 2007; Osguthorpe 2001; Young 2008; Lindbaek 2008). It has been reported that approximately 80% of patients with acute rhinosinusitis improved within 14 days without antibiotics (Ahovuo-Saloranta 2010; Rosenfeld 2007).

A diagnosis of acute bacterial sinusitis may be more likely when:
TWO or MORE MAJOR symptoms are present (ONE of which is nasal obstruction or nasal purulence/discoloured postnasal drainage). Other Major Symptoms: Facial pain/pressure/fullness; hyposomia/anosmia. In addition, the symptoms have not improved after 7 days or have worsened after 5 to 7 days (Desrosiers 2011; SAHP 2004).

Modifying Circumstances	Probable Organism(s)		Antibiotic Choice(s)	Usual Dosage[‡]	Cost per Day
ADULT	**VIRAL**		**No antibiotic indicated**		
	BACTERIAL S. pneumoniae H. influenzae M. catarrhalis S. aureus	*FIRST LINE*	Amoxicillin	500 mg TID	$1.03
		SECOND LINE	Amoxicillin/Clavulanate	500 mg TID or 875 mg BID	$2.00
			Cefuroxime-AX	250-500 mg BID	$1.45 - $2.87
			Cefprozil	250-500 mg BID	$0.86 - $1.70
			Doxycycline	100 mg BID first day then 100 mg once daily	$0.59
			Clarithromycin	500 mg BID or 1000 mg (extended release) once daily	$1.65 - $5.03
			Azithromycin	500 mg daily on first day then 250 mg daily x 4 days	$1.57
			TMP/SMX [4]	2 tabs BID or 1 DS tab BID	$0.08 - $0.24
		THIRD LINE	Levofloxacin [5]	500 mg once daily	$1.37
			Moxifloxacin [5]	400 mg once daily	$6.03

1) Duration of therapy is generally 5-10 days. Another agent may be selected if NO clinical response is seen within 3 days. Note, that successful therapy means good improvement in symptoms at 10 days and NOT complete disappearance of symptoms. **Red Flags for Urgent Referral**: Systemic toxicity, altered mental status, severe headache, swelling of the orbit or change in visual acuity (Desrosiers 2011).
2) **Saline rinses or sprays** (Harvey 2007) **and oral decongestants** may be beneficial.
   Topical decongestants should not be used for more than 3-4 days to avoid rebound congestion.
   Intra-nasal steroids provide positive benefits (reduced severity of symptoms and faster recovery) and may be used alone (i.e., without antibiotics) for the treatment of mild to moderate sinusitis (Desrosiers 2011).
   Antihistamines have not been proven to be effective and thus are not recommended.
3) In chronic sinusitis, antimicrobials do not usually play a major role. For recurrent (≥ 4 episodes per year without signs or symptoms between episodes) or chronic sinusitis (at least 8 to 12 weeks of ≥ two of: mucopurulent drainage, congestion, facial pain/pressure or decreased sense of smell AND documentation of inflammation), exclude the possibility of anatomical abnormalities that may require surgery.
4) Increased pneumococcal and *H. influenzae* resistance rates make TMP/SMX a less desirable agent.
5) Due to the importance of these quinolones for other indications and concern of developing resistance with overuse, these agents need to be held in reserve for severe situations (Adam 2009; Chen 1999).

References: Adam 2009; Ahovuo-Saloranta 2010; Benninger 2006; Bosker 2004; Chen 1999; Desrosiers 2011; de Ferranti 1998; Fairlie 2012; Falagas 2008, 2009; Harvey 2007; Hickner 2001; IDSA 2012; Karageorgopoulos 2008; Klossek 2005; Lindbaek 2008; Luterman 2002; Meltzer 2011; Murray 2000; Randall 2007; Rosenfeld 2007; SAHP 2004; Scheid 2004(a,b); Snow 2001; Williams 1995; Williamson 2007; Wright 2006; Young 2008; Zalmanovici 2009; Zhanel 2002.

TMP/SMX = Trimethoprim / Sulfamethoxazole

Modifying Circumstances	Probable Organism(s)		Antibiotic Choice(s)	Usual Dosage[‡]	Cost per Day

Sinusitis – Children: Acute [1, 2, 3, 4]

CHILDREN	VIRAL		No antibiotic indicated		
	BACTERIAL S. pneumoniae H. influenzae M. catarrhalis	FIRST LINE	Amoxicillin [5]	80 mg/kg/day divided BID or TID (Maximum: 3 g/day)	$0.05/kg
		SECOND LINE	Amoxicillin/Clavulanate [5, 6]	40-80 mg/kg/day amoxicillin divided BID (Maximum: see amoxicillin above)	$0.07 - $0.14/kg
			Cefprozil	30 mg/kg/day divided BID	$0.07/kg
		THIRD LINE	Cefuroxime-AX	30-40 mg/kg/day divided BID	$0.19 - $0.26/kg
			Clarithromycin [7]	15 mg/kg/day divided BID	$0.17/kg
			Azithromycin [7]	10 mg/kg daily on first day then 5 mg/kg daily x 4 days	$0.18/kg
			TMP/SMX [8]	5-10 mg/kg/day trimethoprim divided BID	$0.02 - $0.03/kg

1) For recurrent (≥ 4 episodes per year without signs or symptoms between episodes) or chronic sinusitis (12 weeks or longer of ≥ 2 of: mucopurulent drainage, congestion, facial pain/pressure, or decreased sense of smell AND documentation of inflammation), exclude the possibility of anatomical abnormalities.

2) Two common features – persistent symptoms and severe symptoms – suggest acute bacterial sinusitis.
   Persistent symptoms:
   - Symptoms lasting for longer than 10 days, but less than 30 days, and have not begun to improve. The 10-day mark differentiates simple viral infection from sinusitis.
   - Symptoms include nasal congestion or discharge (any colour) and cough (day and night).
   - Less common include halitosis, facial pain or headache, fatigue and irritability, low-grade fever.
   Severe symptoms: Fever (> 39°C) and purulent nasal discharge.

3) **Approximately 40-60% spontaneous cure rate. NNT = 8 patients for 10 days to achieve short-term benefit (reduced risk of persistent nasal discharge) for one patient; more patients had adverse events with antibiotics (Morris 2002). Hence, amoxicillin is acceptable and preferred for most uncomplicated cases of sinusitis.** Empirically, a 10-14 day course of therapy is recommended (Wald 1992, 1998; O'Brien 1998).

4) Due to lack of evidence on the benefits of antihistamines, decongestants or nasal irrigation in children with acute sinusitus, these agents are NOT recommended (Shaikh 2010).

5) Higher doses have been recommended to eradicate resistant S. pneumoniae (Dowell 1999). A standard 40 mg/kg/day dose could be considered, but not necessarily preferred, in children older than 2 years with no risk factors, including recent antibiotic use, use of daycare, treatment failure, early recurrence or who reside in communities where resistance has been a recognized problem. The 80 mg/kg/day dose is recommended for children 2 years and younger, and/or in daycare, and/or who have had antibiotics in the past 3 months. Maximum amoxicillin dose is 3 g daily (Christian-Kopp 2010).

6) The BID preparation has a lowered clavulanic acid content to improve its tolerance. If less clavulanic acid content is preferred, consider using a combination of amoxicillin 40 mg/kg/day plus amoxicillin/clavulanate 40 mg/kg/day (amoxicillin component) both divided BID (Can Paed Soc 2009).

7) Not appropriate for children < 3 years of age with high fever who may have bacteremia. Pneumococcal meningitis has been reported to develop in young children while taking these medications.

8) Increased pneumococcal and H. influenzae resistance rates make TMP/SMX a less desirable agent.

References: Bosker 2004; Can Paed Soc 2009; Christian-Kopp 2010; Dowell 1999; Hickner 2001; Lusk 2006; IDSA 2012; Morris 2002; O'Brien 1998; Osguthorpe 2001; Pichichero 2008; Ramadan 2005; SAHP 2004; Shaikh 2010; Steele 2005; Wald 1992, 1998.

Acute Bronchitis

In adults, approximately 90% of all cases of acute bronchitis are viral (Gonzales 2000); in children, virtually all cases of acute bronchitis are viral. A number of reviews of the literature do not support routine antibiotic treatment for acute bronchitis (Becker 2000; Bent 1999; Fahey 1998; Gonzales 2000, 2001; MacKay 1996; Orr 1993, Smith 2004; Smucny 1998; Snow 2001).

Emphasize prevention, such as the reduction of risk factors (e.g., smoking cessation and avoidance of second-hand smoke). Current literature does not suggest that antibiotics are beneficial in smokers (MQIC 2008; Linder 2002).

Adults [1, 2, 3]

Modifying Circumstances	Probable Organism(s)	Antibiotic Choice(s)	Usual Dosage	Cost per Day
	Viral (~ 90% of all cases) *Influenza B Influenza A Parainfluenza RSV*	FIRST LINE	**No antibiotic indicated**	

1) Refers to otherwise healthy adults with acute **uncomplicated** bronchitis who do not have underlying lung or heart disease, immunosuppression or bacterial superinfection. Cough usually lasts from 1 to 3 weeks and can present with or without phlegm. Purulent sputum can result from either a viral or bacterial infection. **Ruling out pneumonia is important** and the likelihood is low in the absence of abnormalities in vital signs (heart rate > 100 beats/minute, respiratory rate > 24 breaths/minute, oral temperature > 38°C) and chest examination (focal consolidation – e.g., rales, egophony or fremitus) (Braman 2006; Gonzales 2000, 2001).

2) Increased hydration and humidity are useful in managing cough. If cough suppression is desired, an anti-tussive should be suggested instead of an expectorant preparation. Inhaled bronchodilators have shown a modest effect in protracted cough, specifically in patients with wheezing on physical exam and evidence of airflow obstruction (Becker 2011). Corticosteroids (inhaled or oral) are not generally recommended.

3) Up to 10% of cases of acute bronchitis may be bacterial (*M. pneumonia, C. pneumoniae, B. pertussis*). Cough usually lasts from 1 to 3 weeks and can present with or without phlegm. Prolonged cough (>3 weeks) can occur in up to 50% of cases due to viral infections (Marshall 2011).

References: Attila 2009; Balter 2004; Braman 2006; Becker 2000, 2011; Bent 1999; Butler 2009; Dicpinigaitis 2008; Evans 2002; Fahey 1998; Gonzales 2000, 2001; Linder 2002; MacKay 1996; Marshall 2011; McIssac 2004; MQIC 2008; Orr 1993; Smucny 1998; Steinman 2004; Zhanel 2002.

Children [1, 2]

Modifying Circumstances	Probable Organism(s)	Antibiotic Choice(s)	Usual Dosage	Cost per Day
	Viral 95-100% of all cases of acute bronchitis are viral	FIRST LINE	**No antibiotic indicated**	

1) Fever can be an expected part of a cough illness and may be associated with either a viral or bacterial infection (O'Brien 1998). However, if a child is breathless and/or experiencing tachypnea, consider diagnosis of pneumonia (McCracken 2000).

2) Cough and cold medications are not recommended in the pediatric population (Basco 2009; Health Canada 2008; Taverner 2007).

References: Basco 2009; Health Canada 2008; McCracken 2000; O'Brien 1998; Shields 2008; Taverner 2007.

© 2013 Anti-infective Review Panel

‡ Common oral dosage ranges are provided unless otherwise stated. Consult the drug monograph for details on age and condition-specific dosing. **Page 25**

Modifying Circumstances	Probable Organism(s)		Antibiotic Choice(s)	Usual Dosage‡	Cost per Day

Acute Exacerbations of Chronic Bronchitis (AECB) or Chronic Obstructive Pulmonary Disease (AECOPD) [1, 2, 3, 4]

Presentation with only one of the following cardinal symptoms may not require antibiotics (Anthonisen 1987; GOLD 2010):
1) **Increased dyspnea**
2) **Increased sputum volume**
3) **Increased sputum purulence**

Modifying Circumstances	Probable Organism(s)		Antibiotic Choice(s)	Usual Dosage‡	Cost per Day
SIMPLE [2] (LOW-RISK PATIENTS)	H. influenzae S. pneumoniae M. catarrhalis Haemophilus species	FIRST LINE	Amoxicillin	500 mg TID	$1.03
			Doxycycline	100 mg BID first day then 100 mg once daily	$0.59
			Tetracycline	250-500 mg QID	$0.26 - $0.52
			TMP/SMX	2 tabs BID or 1 DS tab BID	$0.08 - $0.24
			Clarithromycin [4, 5]	500 mg BID or 1000 mg (extended release) once daily	$1.65 - $5.03
			Azithromycin [4, 5]	500 mg on first day then 250 mg daily x 4 days or 500 mg daily x 3 days	$1.57 $2.61
		SECOND LINE	Cefuroxime-AX [4]	500 mg BID	$2.87
			Cefprozil [4]	500 mg BID	$1.70
COMPLICATED [2] (HIGH RISK PATIENTS)	H. influenzae S. pneumoniae M. catarrhalis Haemophilus. species K. pneumoniae	FIRST LINE	Amoxicillin/Clavulanate [4]	500 mg TID or 875 mg BID	$2.00
			Levofloxacin [4, 6]	500 mg once daily x 7 days or 750 mg once daily x 5 days	$1.37 - $6.55
			Moxifloxacin [4, 6]	400 mg once daily	$6.03
PATIENTS AT RISK FOR P. aeruginosa	P. aeruginosa	FIRST LINE	Ciprofloxacin	500-750 mg BID	$1.40 - $2.56

Continued ...

© 2013 Anti-infective Review Panel

TMP/SMX = Trimethoprim / Sulfamethoxazole

Page 26   ‡ Common oral dosage ranges are provided unless otherwise stated. Consult the drug monograph for details on age and condition-specific dosing.

Acute Exacerbations of Chronic Bronchitis (AECB) or Chronic Obstructive Pulmonary Disease (AECOPD)

1) Spirometry (FEV1, FVC not full PFTs) is recommended for determining baseline degree of obstruction as well as selecting and monitoring treatment. **Perform spirometry during exacerbation-free periods.**

   An acute, sustained worsening of baseline symptoms (cough, sputum production/purulence, dyspnea) in those with chronic cough and sputum production (chronic bronchitis) or chronic airflow obstruction (COPD) represents an exacerbation called AECB or AECOPD, respectively. Exacerbations may be purulent or nonpurulent and it has been suggested that antibiotics are only warranted in COPD patients presenting with green (purulent) sputum, with an increase from baseline of either dyspnea or cough (Balter 2004; O'Donnell 2008).

   Approximately 50% of AECB/AECOPD are non-infectious (exposure to allergens and irritants e.g., cigarette smoke, dust, cold air, pollution, chemical irritants) and 50% are infectious (bacterial, viral). Many of the primary viral or non-infectious etiologies may lead to secondary bacterial infections.

   Suggestions to obtain maximum airflow, improve symptoms and prevent future episodes:

   • Counsel patient regarding **smoking cessation and expectation of course of illness**. **Cigarette smoking** is the most common cause of chronic bronchitis and cessation produces dramatic symptomatic benefits.

   • Ensure appropriate doses of bronchodilators and adequate hydration.

   • Maintenance therapy with combination inhaled corticosteroid (ICS)/long-acting beta-agonist (LABA) or long-acting anticholinergic (LAAC) has been shown to decrease the frequency of exacerbations (Calverley 2007; Tashkin 2008).

   • Systemic (oral/parenteral) corticosteroids are of benefit in moderate to severe exacerbations of COPD (in outpatients and AECOPD that require hospitalization) (Aaron 2003; Walters 2009).

2) **Risk Stratification (O'Donnell 2008; Balter 2003):**

   Simple (low risk) patients have chronic bronchitis defined as having chronic cough and sputum production for at least three months for two consecutive years. They usually have mild to moderate impairment of lung function (FEV$_1$> 50% predicted), have four or fewer exacerbations per year and have no significant cardiac disease. Any of the listed antibiotics generally produce good results and the prognosis is excellent.

   Complicated (high risk) patients may have poor underlying lung function (FEV$_1$< 50% predicted) or moderate impairment (FEV$_1$ between 50% and 60% predicted), but demonstrate significant cardiac disease (ischemic heart disease, congestive heart failure) and/or experience four or more exacerbations a year. They may also have other risk factors including use of supplemental oxygen, chronic use of oral steroids or antibiotic use in the past 3 months.

   Patients at risk for pseudomonas infection generally have very poor underlying lung function (FEV$_1$< 35% predicted) or multiple risk factors including frequent exacerbations, chronic oral steroid use, and/or FEV$_1$< 50% predicted. They produce constant purulent sputum and some may have bronchiectasis.

3) **Patients with a relapse within 3 months of using an antibiotic** should receive an alternative class of antibiotic (O'Donnell 2008).

4) **Duration of therapy:** The recommended duration of therapy for mild to moderate AECB may be limited to 5 days, versus 7-10 days, with amoxicillin/clavulanate, 2nd generation cephalosporins (cefuroxime and cefprozil), macrolides and fluoroquinolones (El Moussaoui 2008; Falagas 2008).

5) Prudent use of macrolides will help to preserve this valuable treatment option. Macrolide-resistant *S. pneumoniae* in Canada increased dramatically from 3.7% in 1995 to 19.0% in 2005 (Karlowsky 2009); recent data suggests it is now more than 20% (CBSN 2009). The risk of resistance is greater with longer-acting than with shorter-acting macrolides (azithromycin once daily > clarithromycin BID >> erythromycin QID) (Karlowsky 2009; Malhotra-Kumar 2007; Vanderkooi 2005).

6) Due to the importance of these **quinolones** for other indications and concern of developing resistance with overuse, these agents need to be held in reserve for **severe** situations (Adam 2009; Chen 1999).

References: Adam 2009; Aaron 2003; Adler 2000; Allegra 2005; Anthonisen 1987, 2003; Attila 2009; Aubier 2002; Azithromycin Monograph 2009; Balter 2003, 2004; Bonomo 2002; Burge 2000; Calverley 2007; Chang 2003; Chen 1999; El Moussaoui 2008; Falagas 2008; GOLD 2010; ICSI 2009; Korbila 2009; Mandell 2007; Martinez 2005; Moussaoui 2008; Niewoehner 1999; O'Donnell 2008; Poole 2006; Ram 2006; Resp Review Panel 2007; Sethi 2005; SIGN 2002; Snow 2001; Stockley 2000; Tashkin 2008; Walters 2009; Weiss 2002; Wilson 2008; Woodhead 2005; Zervos 2003; Zhanel 2002.

Modifying Circumstances	Probable Organism(s)	Antibiotic Choice(s)	Usual Dosage‡	Cost per Day

Bronchiectasis: Acute Infective Exacerbations [1, 2, 3]

Modifying Circumstances	Probable Organism(s)	Antibiotic Choice(s)	Usual Dosage‡	Cost per Day
	S. aureus **FIRST** H. influenzae **LINE** [4] S. pneumoniae M. catarrhalis	TMP/SMX	2 tabs BID or 1 DS tab BID **Children:** 5-10 mg/kg/day trimethoprim q12h	$0.08 - $0.24 $0.02 - $0.03/kg
		Amoxicillin/Clavulanate	500 mg TID or 875 mg BID **Children:** 40 mg/kg/day amoxicillin divided q8h	$2.00 $0.07/kg
	P. aeruginosa [1]	Ciprofloxacin	500-750 mg BID **Children:** Not approved, but special cases exist. 20-30 mg/kg/day q12h	$1.40 - $2.56 $0.09 - $0.13/kg

1) Antimicrobial therapy should be directed by cultures. Patients with recent antibiotics exposure and/or cystic fibrosis should be considered at high risk for infection with *Pseudomonas aeruginosa* (Rosen 2006).

2) The most common cause of bronchiectasis in children is cystic fibrosis. A cystic fibrosis patient should not be managed by a family practitioner in isolation; consultation with a specialist is recommended.

3) For suppression of symptoms, long-term low-dose antibiotic therapy may be required for several months. Fluoroquinolones (ciprofloxacin) should not be used in this instance as resistance may build up quickly.

4) Levofloxacin 750 mg once daily for 5 days is a reasonable alternative for non-pseudomonal infection.

References: Barker 2002; Bonomo 2002; Can Paed Soc 2009; Evans 2003; Gibson 2003; King 2007; Rosen 2006; ten Hacken 2007; Tsang 1999; Woodhead 2005.

TMP/SMX = Trimethoprim / Sulfamethoxazole

‡ Common oral dosage ranges are provided unless otherwise stated. Consult the drug monograph for details on age and condition-specific dosing.

Community-acquired Pneumonia

General Statements:

The following treatment tables are generally for empiric treatment and are based primarily on the references below, the consensus of experts, clinical experience, and in vitro activity. We have attempted to allow maximum flexibility for the prescriber through acknowledgement of the varying approaches suggested by different guidelines and clinical opinion. Please note that at anytime empiric therapy can be adjusted once more information becomes available regarding the etiologic agent.

- Physicians are encouraged to be aware of **local antimicrobial susceptibility patterns** to facilitate antibiotic selection.
- It is important to obtain a **patient's antibiotic history**. Review antibiotics prescribed for any type of infection in the previous 3 months; if there has been significant exposure to a particular antibiotic class, then select an agent from an alternate class, particularly for macrolides and fluoroquinolones (Mandell 2007).
- **Site of Care Decision – To Hospitalize or Not?** Severity of illness-score can be used to identify patients who should be hospitalized. Criteria scores should always be supplemented with determination of subjective factors (e.g., reliability to take oral medications and availability of out-patient support) (Niederman 2009).
  CRB-65 criteria: Confusion (new onset disorientation), **R**espiratory rate (> 30 breaths/minute), low **B**lood pressure (<90 SBP and/or < 60 DBP), **A**ge > 65 score. Score 1 point for each criterion. If CRB-65 score is ≥ 3, admit urgently. If score is 2, same day assessment in secondary care. If score is 0-1, treatment at home may be appropriate depending on clinical judgement and available support (Bauer 2006). Of note, in community settings, CRB-65 may over-predict 30-day mortality risk (McNally 2010).
- **Fluoroquinolones** should be reserved for treatment failures, comorbidities with recent antibiotic use, allergies or documented infections with highly drug-resistant pneumococci. This is due to their broad-spectrum of activity, concerns over the rapid emergence of fluoroquinolone-resistance pneumococci and *C.difficile*-associated disease (Owens 2008). Acquisition of a respiratory infection in a hospital or nursing home is a significant risk factor for infection with fluoroquinolone-resistant pneumococci (Adam 2009; Chen 1999; Mandell 2007; Mills 2009).
- **Macrolide-resistant** *S. pneumoniae* in Canada increased dramatically from 3.7% in 1995 to 19.0% in 2005 (Karlowsky 2009); recent data suggests it is now more than 20% (CBSN 2009). Macrolide use is the single most important driver of this and has been shown to increase the colonization of macrolide-resistant *S. pneumoniae* by 50%. The risk of resistance is greater with longer-acting than with shorter-acting macrolides (azithromycin once daily > clarithromycin BID >> erythromycin QID). Thus, the risk associated with previous use of azithromycin is greater than with use of other macrolides (Malhotra-Kumar 2007; Vanderkooi 2005).
- **Duration of therapy** depends on various factors (e.g., clinical presentation, co-morbidities, age, the drug selected, etc.) and typically varies from 7-14 days. There is good evidence that shorter courses of therapy are equally effective in ambulatory patients. Patients should be treated for a minimum of 5 days, be afebrile for 48-72 hours, and otherwise clinically stable before discontinuing therapy (Li 2007; Mandell 2007; Scalera 2007).

References: Adam 2009; Armitage 2007; Bauer 2006; CBSN 2009; Chen 1999; File 2009; Grant 2009; Karlowsky 2009; Li 2007; Lim 2009; Malhotra-Kumar 2007; Mandell 2007; McNally 2010; Mills 2009; Niederman 2009; Owens 2008; Scalera 2007; Vanderkooi 2005; Vardakas 2008.

Modifying Circumstances	Probable Organism(s)		Antibiotic Choice(s)	Usual Dosage‡	Cost per Day

Pneumonia – Adult: Community-acquired, mild to moderate [1,2]

Outpatient without comorbidity / modifying factors [3]

Modifying Circumstances	Probable Organism(s)		Antibiotic Choice(s)	Usual Dosage‡	Cost per Day
	S. pneumoniae	FIRST LINE	Amoxicillin [2]	1 g TID	$2.05
	M. pneumoniae		Erythromycin	500 mg QID	$1.47
	C. pneumoniae		Clarithromycin	500mg BID or 1000 mg (extended release) once daily	$1.65 - $5.03
			Azithromycin	500 mg daily on first day then 250 mg daily x 4 days or 500 mg daily x 3 days	$1.57 / $2.61
		SECOND LINE	Doxycycline	100 mg BID first day then 100 mg once daily	$0.59

Outpatient with comorbidity/modifying factors

Modifying Circumstances	Probable Organism(s)		Antibiotic Choice(s)	Usual Dosage‡	Cost per Day
Comorbidity [3] or Antibiotic within last 3 months	S. pneumoniae M. pneumoniae C. pneumoniae H. influenzae	FIRST LINE	Amoxicillin [2]	1 g TID	$2.05
			Amoxicillin/Clavulanate	500 mg TID or 875 mg BID	$2.00
			Cefuroxime-AX	500 mg BID	$2.86
			Cefprozil	500 mg BID	$1.70
			ANY ONE of the beta-lactam agents above PLUS ONE of the following:		
			Clarithromycin	500 mg BID or 1000 mg (extended release) once daily	$1.65 - $5.03
			Azithromycin	500 mg daily on first day then 250 mg daily x 4 days	$1.57
			Doxycycline	100 mg BID first day then 100 mg once daily	$0.59
			OR any ONE of the following:		
			Levofloxacin [4]	750 mg once daily x 5 days	$2.57 - $6.55
			Moxifloxacin [4]	400 mg once daily	$6.03
SUSPECTED ASPIRATION [5]	Polymicrobial Oral anaerobes Gram -ve bacilli	FIRST LINE	Amoxicillin/Clavulanate	500 mg TID or 875 mg BID	$2.00
			Clindamycin	300-450 mg QID	$1.77 - $2.66

Continued ...

‡ Common oral dosage ranges are provided unless otherwise stated. Consult the drug monograph for details on age and condition-specific dosing.

Pneumonia – Adult: Community-acquired, mild to moderate

1) **It is important to obtain a patient's antibiotic history.** Review antibiotics prescribed for any type of infection in the previous 3 months; if there has been significant exposure to a particular antibiotic class, then consider selecting an alternate class. In regions with a high rate (> 25%) of macrolide resistant *S. pneumoniae*, consider the use of alternative agents, including in those patients without comorbidities (Mandell 2007).

   Duration of therapy depends on various factors (e.g., clinical presentation, comorbidities, age, the drug selected, etc.) and typically varies from 7-14 days; however, there is good evidence that shorter courses of therapy are equally effective in ambulatory patients. Patients should be treated for a minimum of 5 days, be afebrile for 48-72 hrs, and otherwise clinically stable before discontinuing therapy (Li 2007; Mandell 2007; Scalera 2007). An exception is azithromycin 500 mg which may be used for 3 days in outpatients without comorbidity.

2) Amoxicillin 1000 mg TID is active against 90-95% of *S. pneumoniae* and can be considered for patients over 50 years of age where *Mycoplasma* infection is less likely (Mandell 2007; Mills 2005).

3) Comorbidity/modifying factors: hospitalization in the past 3 months and/or chronic heart, lung, liver or renal disease, diabetes mellitus, alcoholism, malignancies, asplenia, immunosuppression.

4) Fluoroquinolones should be reserved for treatment failures, comorbidities with recent antibiotic use, allergies or documented infections with highly drug-resistant pneumococci (Adam 2009; Chen 1999; Mandell 2007). This is due to their broad-spectrum of activity, concerns over the rapid emergence of fluoroquinolone-resistance pneumococci and *C.difficile*-associated disease (Owens 2008).

5) Anaerobic coverage is clearly indicated only in the classic aspiration pleuropulmonary syndrome in patients with a history of loss of consciousness as a result of alcohol/drug overdose or after seizures in patients with concomitant gingival disease or esophageal motility disorders. Consider aspiration pneumonia in patients with difficulties swallowing who show clinical signs of a lower respiratory tract infection (Mandell 2007; Woodhead 2005).

References: Adam 2009; Armitage 2007; Arnold 2007; Bartlett 2000; BTS 2004; Daneman 2006, 2008; Dunbar 2003; File 2009; Fogarty 2003; Gotfried 2002; Grenier 2011; Hadberg 2002; Li 2007; Lim 2009; Mandell 2007; McCusker 2003; Owens 2008; Paris 2008; Scalara 2007; Vanderkooi 2005; Van Rensberg 2002; Vardakas 2008; Woodhead 2005; Zhanel 2002.

Modifying Circumstances	Probable Organism(s)	Antibiotic Choice(s)	Usual Dosage‡	Cost per Day

Pneumonia – Long-Term Care: Mild to moderate [1]

S. pneumoniae **FIRST** H. influenzae **LINE** Gram -ve bacilli S. aureus Legionella spp. C pneumoniae		**Amoxicillin**	1 g TID	$2.05
		Amoxicillin/Clavulanate	500 mg TID or 875 mg BID	$2.00
		Cefuroxime-AX	500 mg BID	$2.86
		Cefprozil	500 mg BID	$1.70

ANY ONE of the beta-lactam agents above
PLUS ONE of the following:

		Clarithromycin	500 mg BID or 1000 mg (extended release) once daily	$1.65 - $5.03
		Azithromycin	500 mg daily on first day then 250 mg daily x 4 days	$1.57
		Doxycycline	100 mg BID first day then 100 mg once daily	$0.59

OR any ONE of the following:

		Levofloxacin [2]	750 mg once daily x 5 days	$2.57 - $6.55
		Moxifloxacin [2]	400 mg once daily	$6.03

1) For suspected aspiration, see page 30.
2) Patients from nursing homes and/or with recent exposure to hospitals are more likely to be infected with fluoroquinolone resistant pathogens. Consult local antimicrobial susceptibility patterns to facilitate antibiotic selection. For example, residents of nursing homes presenting to hospitals with laboratory-confirmed pneumococcal disease having a rate of resistance, or partial resistance, to levofloxacin of 4%. Thus, in such regions, fluoroquinolone monotherapy is not recommended for infections of the respiratory tract in nursing home residents (TIBDN 2009; UHN 2009).

References: Arnold 2007; Bonomo 2002; BTS 2004; Dunbar 2003; Furman 2004; Hutt 2002; Gotfried 2002; Grenier 2011; Lim 2009; Loeb 1999, 2003, 2006; Mandell 2007; Marik 2003; Marrie 2002; Mills 2009; Mylotte 2002; Naughton 2000; Rotstein 2008; Solh 2004; TIBDN 2009; UHN 2009; Vardakas 2008; Zhanel 2002.

Modifying Circumstances	Probable Organism(s)	Antibiotic Choice(s)	Usual Dosage‡	Cost per Day

Pneumonia – Adult: Severe (requiring hospitalization)
Community-acquired or Long-Term Care [1, 2, 3]

Modifying Circumstances	Probable Organism(s)	Antibiotic Choice(s)	Usual Dosage‡	Cost per Day
PATIENT ON MEDICAL WARD	S. pneumoniae **FIRST** M. pneumoniae **LINE** C. pneumoniae H. influenzae Legionella spp.	Cefotaxime IV	1 - 2 g q8h	$27.60 - $55.20
		Ceftriaxone IV	1 - 2 g q24h	$12.50 - $24.14
		Amoxicillin	1 g TID	$2.05
		Amoxicillin/Clavulanate	500 mg TID or 875 mg BID	$2.00
		ANY ONE of the beta-lactam agents above PLUS ONE of the following:		
		Clarithromycin	500 mg BID or 1000 mg (extended release) once daily	$1.65 - $5.03
		Azithromycin	500 mg daily on first day then 250 mg daily x 4 days	$1.57
		Doxycycline	100 mg BID first day then 100 mg once daily	$0.59
		OR any ONE of the following:		
		Levofloxacin PO/IV [4]	PO: 750 mg once daily x 7-14 days	$2.57 - $6.55
			IV: 500 - 750 mg q24h	IV: $23.80-$30.97
		Moxifloxacin PO/IV [4]	400 mg once daily x 7-14 days	PO: $6.03 IV: $34.00

1) **Site of Care Decision - To Hospitalize or Not?** Severity of illness-scores can be used to identify community-acquired pneumonia patients who may be candidates for outpatient treatment. Criteria scores should always be supplemented with determination of subjective factors (e.g., reliability to take oral medications and availability of outpatient support) (Niederman 2009).

   CRB-65 criteria: Confusion (new onset disorientation), **R**espiratory rate ($\geq$ 30 breaths/minute), low **B**lood pressure (<90 SBP and/or <60 DBP), **A**ge $\geq$ 65 years. Score 1 point for each criterion. If CRB-65 score, $\geq$ 3 admit urgently. If score is 2, same day assessment in secondary care. If score is 0-1, treatment at home may be appropriate depending on clinical judgement and available support (Bauer 2006). Of note, in community settings, CRB-65 may over-predict 30-day mortality risk (McNally 2010).

2) Hospitalized patients may use oral antibiotics if they are hemodynamically stable and do not require intensive care, have a normal functioning GI tract and the drug being used does not have a history of causing GI intolerance, and are closely monitored during the first 48 hours of treatment. Patients who are started on IV therapy should be assessed for step-down to oral therapy as soon as they can tolerate oral medications.

3) It is important to obtain a patient's antibiotic history. Review antibiotics prescribed for any type of infection in the previous 3 months; if there has been significant exposure to a particular antibiotic class, then consider selecting from an alternate class (Mandell 2007).

4) Patients from nursing homes and/or with recent exposure to hospitals are more likely to be infected with fluoroquinolone resistant pathogens.

References: Bauer 2006; Bonomo 2002; BTS 2004; Dunbar 2003; File 2009; Fine 1997; Gotfried 2002; Lim 2003, 2009; Mandell 2007; McNally 2010; Niederman 2009; Rotstein 2008; UHN 2009; West 2003; Zhanel 2002.

© 2013 Anti-infective Review Panel

‡ Common oral dosage ranges are provided unless otherwise stated. Consult the drug monograph for details on age and condition-specific dosing. **Page 33**

Pneumonia – Adult: Severe (Intensive Care Unit) [1, 2, 3]
Community-acquired or Long-term Care

Modifying Circumstances	Probable Organism(s)	Antibiotic Choice(s)	Usual Dosage‡	Cost per Day
WHEN P. AERUGINOSA IS NOT A CONCERN	S. pneumoniae S. aureus Legionella spp. Gram -ve bacilli H. influenzae	**FIRST LINE** Cefotaxime IV	1 - 2 g q6-8h	$27.60 - $55.20
		Ceftriaxone IM/IV	1 - 2 g q24h	$12.50 - $24.14
		ANY ONE of the above PLUS ONE of the following:		
		Clarithromycin	500 mg BID or 1000 mg (extended release) once daily	$1.65 - $5.03
		Azithromycin PO/IV	500 mg q24h	PO: $4.93 IV: varies
		Levofloxacin PO/IV [4]	PO: 750 mg once daily x 7-14 days IV: 750 mg q24h	PO: $2.57 - $6.55 IV: varies
		Moxifloxacin PO/IV [4]	400 mg once daily	PO: $6.03 IV: varies
	BETA-LACTAM ALLERGY	**Any ONE Fluoroquinolone above PLUS**		
		Clindamycin PO/IV	PO: 300 - 450 mg QID IV: 600 mg q8h	$1.77 - $2.66 IV: varies

1) Criteria for severe pneumonia requiring ICU admission include: arterial hypoxemia despite oxygen supplementation, respiratory rate more than 30 per minute, need for ventilator support, and shock (DBP < 60 mmHg or SBP < 90 mmHg).

2) Review antibiotics prescribed for any type of infection in the previous 3 months; if there has been significant exposure to a particular class of agents, then consider selecting an alternative class of antibiotic agent (Mandell 2007).

3) Healthcare-associated pneumonia (HCAP) is defined as pneumonia that occurs in a non-hospitalized patient with extensive healthcare contact, as defined by one or more of the following (IDSA-Craven 2005): IV therapy, wound care, or IV chemotherapy within the prior 30 days; residence in a nursing home or other LTC; hospitalization in an acute care hospital for two or more days within the prior 90 days or attendance at a hospital or hemodialysis clinic within the prior 30 days. It has been suggested that 'HCAP' pneumonia occurring in non-ambulatory residents of nursing homes and other LTC facilities be treated in a similar manner to hospital-acquired (or nosocomial) pneumonia since it is more likely to be caused by resistant pathogens, however, significant heterogeneity among this group makes a blanket approach to treatment problematic. Certain patients whose conditions are included in the designation of HCAP are better served by management in accordance with standard CAP guidelines with concern for specific pathogens (Mandell 2007). The HCAP category continues to be a subject of controversy since it results in overtreatment without any evidence for improved outcomes (Ewig 2012).

4) Patients from nursing homes and/or with recent exposure to hospitals are more likely to be infected with fluoroquinolone-resistant pathogens.

References: Bonfiglio 2001; BTS 2004; Dunbar 2003; Ewig 2012; File 2009; IDSA-Craven 2005; Lim 2009; Mandell 2007; Rotstein 2008; Vanderkooi 2005; Vardakas 2008; West 2003.

© 2013 Anti-infective Review Panel

Page 34   ‡ Common oral dosage ranges are provided unless otherwise stated. Consult the drug monograph for details on age and condition-specific dosing.

Pneumonia – Adult: Severe (Intensive Care Unit)[1, 2]

Community-acquired or Long-term Care - Pseudomonas an Issue

Modifying Circumstances	Probable Organism(s)	Antibiotic Choice(s)		Usual Dosage‡	Cost per Day
STRUCTURAL LUNG DISEASE (i.e., bronchiectasis or cystic fibrosis where *P. aeruginosa* may be suspected[3])	*P. aeruginosa*[3] *S. pneumoniae* *S. aureus* *Legionella spp.* Gram -ve bacilli *H. influenzae*	**FIRST LINE**	Ciprofloxacin PO	750 mg BID	$2.56
			Ciprofloxacin IV	400 mg q8-12h	
			ONE of the above PLUS ONE of the following:		
			Cefepime IV	1 - 2 g q8h	IV costs vary according to jurisdiction and/or contract pricing.
			Ceftazidime IV	1 - 2 g q8h	
			Piperacilin/Tazobactam IV	4.5 g / 0.5 g q8h	
			Imipenem/Cilastatin IV	500 mg q6h	
			Meropenem IV	1 g q8h	
		SECOND LINE	Triple therapy with an antipseudomonal ß-lactam (e.g., cefepime or ceftazidime, piperacillin-tazobactam, imipenem or meropenem) plus aminoglycoside plus a fluoroquinolone.		

1) Criteria for severe pneumonia requiring ICU admission include: arterial hypoxemia despite oxygen supplementation; respiratory rate more than 30 breaths per minute; need for ventilator support; and shock (DBP < 60 mmHg or SBP < 90 mmHg).

2) Review antibiotics prescribed for any type of infection in the previous 3 months; if there has been significant exposure to a particular class of agents, then consider selecting an alternative class of antibiotic agent. If CA-MRSA is suspected, add vancomycin to therapy (Mandell 2007).

3) If *P. aeruginosa* is cultured, a combination of an aminoglycoside plus an anti-pseudomonal ß-lactam (e.g., cefepime, ceftazidime, piperacillin, imipenem, meropenem) can be used. Risk factors for infection with *P. aeruginosa* include severe underlying bronchopulmonary disease (e.g., bronchiectasis), alcoholism, frequent courses of antibiotics (> 4 courses/year), recent antibiotic use (past 3 months), chronic oral steroid therapy or history of recent hospital stay, especially ICU.

References: Bonfiglio 2001; BTS 2004; Ewig 2012; IDSA 2005-Craven; Lim 2009; Low 2008; Mandell 2007; Rotstein 2008; Woodhead 2005.

© 2013 Anti-infective Review Panel

‡ Common oral dosage ranges are provided unless otherwise stated. Consult the drug monograph for details on age and condition-specific dosing. **Page 35**

Modifying Circumstances	Probable Organism(s)		Antibiotic Choice(s)	Usual Dosage‡	Cost per Day

Pneumonia – Children: Outpatients [1, 2, 3, 4]

Modifying Circumstances	Probable Organism(s)		Antibiotic Choice(s)	Usual Dosage‡	Cost per Day
1 - 3 MONTHS OF AGE	For this age group (1-3 months), consult a specialist. Initial <u>outpatient</u> treatment is NOT recommended due to the complexity of the problem in very young infants.				
3 MONTHS TO 5 YEARS	RSV Other viruses		**No antibiotic indicated**		
(Preschool)	S. pneumoniae S. aureus	*FIRST LINE*	**Amoxicillin**	80 mg/kg/day divided TID for 7-10 days	$0.05/kg
	Group A Strep. H. influenzae		**Amoxicillin/Clavulanate**	80 mg/kg/day amoxicillin divided BID	$0.14/kg
	C. trachomatis M. pneumoniae C. pneumoniae	*β-LACTAM ALLERGY[5]*	**Erythromycin estolate/ base**	40 mg/kg/day divided BID, TID or QID for 7-10 days	$0.04 - $0.36/kg
			Clarithromycin	15 mg/kg/day divided BID for 7-10 days	$0.17/kg
			Azithromycin	10 mg/kg/day on first day then 5 mg/kg/day x 4 days	$0.18/kg
5 - 18 YEARS **(School-age)**	M. pneumoniae C. pneumoniae S. pneumoniae	*FIRST LINE[5]*	**Erythromycin estolate/ base**	40 mg/kg/day divided BID, TID or QID for 7-10 days (Maximum: 4 g/day)	$0.04 - $0.36/kg
	Influenza A or B Adenovirus Other respiratory viruses		**Clarithromycin**	15 mg/kg/day divided BID for 7-10 days (Maximum: 1 g/day)	$0.17/kg
			Azithromycin	10 mg/kg/day on first day then 5 mg/kg/day x 4 days (Maximum: 1.5 g/5-day)	$0.18/kg
			Doxycycline	2-4 mg/kg/day divided BID (> 8 years old) (Maximum: 200 mg/day)	$0.68/kg

1) Viruses are the most frequent cause of pneumonia in the first 5 years of a child's life. In children 3 months to 5 years most bacterial pneumonias are due to *S. pneumoniae*; *H. influenza* type b has almost disappeared because of vaccination. In children greater than 5 years most bacterial pneumonias are due to *M. pneumoniae* and *C. pneumoniae*. Clinical improvement should be seen within 48 hours with bacterial pneumonia, however this often takes longer with viral pneumonia (Can Paed Soc-Le Saux 2011).

2) Most children can be managed as outpatients. **Consider hospitalization** if: Age less than 1 month, toxic appearance, severe respiratory distress, oxygen requirement, dehydration, vomiting, no response to appropriate oral antimicrobial therapy, immunocompromised host, hypotension or any evidence of an empyema or lung abscess (Low 2003).

3) The routine use of chest radiography for children with wheezing but without fever should be discouraged (Mathews 2009).

4) Review antibiotics prescribed for any type of infection in the previous 3 months; if there has been significant exposure to a particular class of agents, then consider selecting an alternative class of antibiotic agent (Mandell 2007).

5) Safety and effectiveness of azithromycin and clarithromycin in pediatric pneumonia has not been demonstrated in children less than 6 months of age (CPS 2012).

References: Bennett 2011; Bowen 2013; BTS 2011; Can Paed Soc-Le Saux 2011; CPS 2012; Grant 2009; IDSA 2011; Jadavji 1997; Low 2003; Mandell 2007; Mathews 2009; McIntosh 2002; Ostapchuk 2004; Powell 2006.

Modifying Circumstances	Probable Organism(s)	Antibiotic Choice(s)	Usual Dosage[‡]	Cost per Day

Pneumonia – Children: Hospitalized [1, 2]

Modifying Circumstances	Probable Organism(s)	Antibiotic Choice(s)	Usual Dosage[‡]	Cost per Day
1 - 3 MONTHS OF AGE	For this age group (1-3 months), consult a specialist.			
3 MONTHS TO 5 YEARS	RSV Other viruses	**No antibiotic indicated**		
(Preschool)	S. pneumoniae **FIRST** S. aureus **LINE** Group A. Strep. H. influenzae M. pneumoniae C. pneumoniae	Ampicillin IV [3] Cefuroxime IV [3] Ceftriaxone IM/IV Cefotaxime IV	150-200 mg/kg/day divided q6h 150 mg/kg/day divided q8h 75-100 mg/kg/day divided q12-24h 200 mg/kg/day divided q6h	IV costs vary according to jurisdiction and/or contract pricing.
		One of the above ± ONE of the following (if atypical organism(s) suspected):		
		Erythromycin PO	40 mg/kg/day divided QID	$0.04 - $0.36/kg
		Clarithromycin [4]	15 mg/kg/day divided BID	$0.17/kg
		Azithromycin PO/IV [4]	10 mg/kg/day on first day then 5 mg/kg/day x 4 days	$0.18/kg
5 - 18 YEARS **(School-age)**	S. pneumoniae **FIRST** M. pneumoniae **LINE** C. pneumoniae Influenza A or B Adenovirus Other respiratory viruses	Ampicillin IV [3] Cefuroxime IV [3] Ceftriaxone IM/IV Cefotaxime IV	150-200 mg/kg/day divided q6h (Maximum: 8 g/day) 150 mg/kg/day divided q8h (Maximum: 4.5 g/day) 75-100 mg/kg/day divided q12-24h (Maximum: 2g/day) 200 mg/kg/day divided q6h (Maximum: 8 g/day)	IV costs vary according to jurisdiction and/or contract pricing.
		One of the above PLUS ONE of the following:		
		Erythromycin PO	40 mg/kg/day divided QID (Maximum: 4 g/day)	$0.04 - $0.36/kg
		Clarithromycin [4]	15 mg/kg/day divided BID (Maximum: 1 g/day)	$0.17/kg
		Azithromycin PO/IV [4]	10 mg/kg/day on first day then 5 mg/kg/day x 4 days (Maximum: 1.5 g/5-day)	$0.18/kg

1) Consider hospitalization when less than one month of age, toxic appearance, severe respiratory distress, oxygen requirement, dehydration, vomiting, no response to appropriate oral antimicrobial therapy, immunocompromised host. Add vancomycin or linezolid to antibiotic regimen if suspected CA-MRSA.

2) Viruses are the most frequent cause of pneumonia in the first 5 years of a child's life. In children 3 months to 5 years most bacterial pneumonias are due to S. pneumoniae; H. influenza type b has almost disappeared because of vaccination. In children greater than 5 years most bacterial pneumonias are due to M. pneumoniae and C. pneumoniae. Clinical improvement should be seen within 48 hours with bacterial pneumonia, however improvement often takes longer with viral pneumonia (Can Paed Soc-Le Saux 2011).

3) Ampicillin or cefuroxime are options for non-severe pneumonia and may be given orally where feasible.

4) Safety and effectiveness of azithromycin and clarithromycin in pediatric pneumonia has not been demonstrated in children less than 6 months of age (CPS 2012).

References: Bennett 2011; BTS 2011; Can Paed Soc-Le Saux 2011; CPS 2012; Esposito 2012 (a, b); IDSA 2011; Jadavji 1997; Low 2003, 2008; Mandell 2007; McIntosh 2002; Ostapchuk 2004; Principi 2011; Rojas 2006; Sick Kids 2012/2013.

© 2013 Anti-infective Review Panel

‡ Common oral dosage ranges are provided unless otherwise stated. Consult the drug monograph for details on age and condition-specific dosing. **Page 37**

Modifying Circumstances	Probable Organism(s)		Antibiotic Choice(s)	Usual Dosage‡	Cost per Day

Pertussis (Whooping Cough) [1, 2, 3, 4]

Modifying Circumstances	Probable Organism(s)		Antibiotic Choice(s)	Usual Dosage‡	Cost per Day
ADULT AND CHILDREN	*B. pertussis*	**FIRST LINE**	Erythromycin (for adult)	1 - 2 g/day divided BID, TID or QID	$0.18 - $0.36
			Erythromycin estolate (for children)	**Children:** 30 - 40 mg/kg/day divided q6-8h for 7 days [5]	$0.03 - $0.04/kg
			Clarithromycin	250 - 500 mg BID	$0.82 - $1.65
				Children: 15 mg/kg/day divided BID	$0.17/kg
			Azithromycin	500 mg daily on first day then 250 mg daily x 4 days	$1.57
				Children: 10 mg/kg/day on first day then 5 mg/kg/day x 4 days	$0.18/kg
		SECOND LINE	TMP/SMX	2 tabs BID or 1 DS tab BID	$0.08 - $0.24
				Children: 5 - 10 mg/kg/day divided BID	$0.02 - $0.03/kg

1) For current Canadian pertussis vaccination schedules see: www.phac-aspc.gc.ca. Maintenance of high vaccination rates is the most effective way to prevent pertussis. Minimizing exposure of infants is also effective. Individuals spontaneously clear pertussis from their nasopharynx within 3-4 weeks of cough onset in 80-90% of cases. Untreated and unvaccinated infants can remain culture positive for > 6 weeks.

2) Suspect pertussis in individuals with paroxysmal cough of any duration; cough with inspiratory whoop; cough ending in vomiting or gagging or associated with apnea with no other known cause (NACI 2006).

3) Notify the Medical Officer of Health and consult with public health authorities and ensure that all household contacts, regardless of age and immunization status, are offered chemoprophylaxis; same drug regimen as for active case - see table above. Administration of antibiotics for treatment of whooping cough is effective for nasopharynx eradication of *B. pertussis,* but does not alter subsequent clinical course of the infection and has not demonstrated a benefit in terms of averting clinical symptoms of infection. However, the grave effects of pertussis infection in vulnerable patients makes prophylaxis imperative in infants < 1 year old or patients in 3rd trimester of pregnancy who reside in the same household or have been in a confined space with the index case (Altunaiji 2007; NACI 2006; PHAC 2012; Tiwari 2005). Chemoprophylaxis should be implemented as soon as possible; efficacy is related to early implementation and is unlikely to be of any benefit after 21 days have elapsed since the first contact.

4) Duration of therapy is usually 5 to 7 days, depending on the agent. However, antibiotic therapy started three weeks after the onset of symptoms is of no benefit since the organism has already been spontaneously cleared from the nasopharynx. The patient is usually considered infectious until 3 weeks after the onset of cough (without therapy), or until 5 days after the start of therapy.

5) The 7 day course of treatment recommendation is based on a study by Halperin (1997).

References: Am Acad Ped 2006; Altunaiji 2007; Bace 1999; CDC 2005, 2011, 2012, 2013; De Serres 1995; Frumkin 2012; Halperin 1997; Lebel 2001; NACI 2006, 2007, 2013; National Consensus Conference on Pertussis 2002; PHAC 2012; Pichichero 2003; Tiwari 2005.

© 2013 Anti-infective Review Panel   TMP/SMX = Trimethoprim / Sulfamethoxazole

Page 38   ‡ Common oral dosage ranges are provided unless otherwise stated. Consult the drug monograph for details on age and condition-specific dosing.

Skin Infections

Modifying Circumstances	Probable Organism(s)	Antibiotic Choice(s)		Usual Dosage‡	Cost per Day

Impetigo & Bullous Impetigo – Adult [1, 2, 3, 4]

Modifying Circumstances	Probable Organism(s)	Antibiotic Choice(s)		Usual Dosage‡	Cost per Day
	S. aureus Group A Strep.	FIRST LINE	Topical therapy in less severe / localized cases:		
			Mupirocin 2% [5] ung/cream	Apply sparingly TID	15 g ung: $5.33 15 g cr: $7.85
			Fusidic acid 2% [5] ung/cream	Apply sparingly TID - QID. If covered with occlusive dressing, then daily or BID.	15 g: $8.74
			Systemic antibiotics for significant soft tissue infections or during community outbreaks:		
			Cloxacillin	250-500 mg QID	$0.74 - $1.40
			Cephalexin	250-500 mg QID	$0.90 - $1.80
		SECOND LINE	Erythromycin	1 g/day divided BID, TID or QID	$0.18
			Clarithromycin	250 mg BID	$0.82
			Azithromycin	500 mg daily on first day then 250 mg daily x 4 days	$1.57
			Clindamycin	150-300 mg QID	$0.89 - $1.77

1) The majority of infections of mild severity can be treated topically; the decision of how to treat depends on the number of lesions, their location (face, eyelid or mouth), and the need to limit the spread of infection to others (Stevens 2005). Use topical therapy when infection is limited and localized (i.e., two to three small areas). Consider systemic therapy if infection is widespread, if patient is immunocompromised, has valvular heart disease, fever, constitutional symptoms suggesting bacteremia, has not improved from topical therapy within 24-48 hours and/or MRSA is a possibility. In multiple drug allergy, minocycline 100 mg BID is an alternative.

2) Outbreaks should not be treated with topical therapy; consider performing cultures if complicated and/or during epidemics. Duration of treatment generally 7-10 days (Cole 2007; Stevens 2005).

3) **Recurrent impetigo:** the most common underlying factor is S. aureus carriage in the anterior nares or perineum. Evaluate by culturing and if positive, treat topically with mupirocin or fusidic acid 2-3 times daily for 2-3 days. Another common cause of recurrent impetigo is secondary bacterial impetiginization of underlying dermatoses, such as eczema or psoriasis. In these cases, the impetigo still needs therapy with antibacterials, but the underlying disease should be treated as well.

4) Bullous impetigo is due to S. aureus with production of epidermolytic toxin locally.

5) It has not been shown necessary to remove the crusts before application of fusidic acid or mupirocin. Duration of therapy is generally 5-7 days (Cole 2007).

References: Brown 2003; Cole 2007; George 2003; Koning 2004; Leyden 2003; Stevens 2005.

© 2013 Anti-infective Review Panel

‡ Common oral dosage ranges are provided unless otherwise stated. Consult the drug monograph for details on age and condition-specific dosing. **Page 41**

Impetigo & Bullous Impetigo – Children [1, 2, 3, 4]

Modifying Circumstances	Probable Organism(s)	Antibiotic Choice(s)	Usual Dosage‡	Cost per Day
	S. aureus Group A Strep. **FIRST LINE**	**Topical therapy in less severe / localized cases:**		
		Mupirocin 2% ung/cream [5]	Apply sparingly TID	15 g ung: $5.33 15 g cr: $7.85
		Fusidic acid 2% ung/cream [5]	Apply sparingly TID - QID. If covered with occlusive dressing, then daily or BID.	15 g: $8.74
		Systemic antibiotics for significant soft tissue infections or during community outbreaks:		
		Cephalexin	50-100 mg/kg/day divided QID	$0.06 - $0.13/kg
	SECOND LINE	Erythromycin estolate	30-40 mg/kg/day divided QID	$0.03 - $0.04/kg
		Clarithromycin	15 mg/kg/day divided BID	$0.17/kg
		Azithromycin	10 mg/kg daily on first day then 5 mg/kg daily x 4 days	$0.18/kg
		Clindamycin	10-20 mg/kg/day divided TID or QID	$0.07 - $0.14/kg
	THIRD LINE	Cloxacillin	50 mg/kg/day divided QID	$0.09/kg

1) The majority of infections of mild severity can be treated topically. Use topical therapy when infection is limited and localized (i.e., two to three small areas). Consider systemic therapy if infection is widespread, if patient is immunocompromised, has valvular heart disease, fever, constitutional symptoms suggesting bacteremia or has not improved from topical therapy within 24-48 hours and/or possible MRSA.

2) Outbreaks should not be treated with topical therapy; consider performing cultures if complicated and/or during epidemics. Duration of treatment generally 7-10 days (Cole 2007; Oumeish 2000; Stevens 2005).

3) **Recurrent impetigo:** the most common underlying factor is S. aureus carriage in the anterior nares or perineum. Evaluate by culturing and if positive, treat topically with mupirocin or fusidic acid 2-3 times daily for 2-3 days. Another common cause of recurrent impetigo is secondary bacterial impetiginization of underlying dermatoses such as eczema or psoriasis. In these cases, the impetigo still needs therapy with antibacterials, but the underlying disease should be treated as well.

4) Bullous impetigo is due to S. aureus with production of epidermolytic toxin locally.

5) It has not been shown necessary to remove the crusts before application of fusidic acid or mupirocin. Duration of therapy generally 5-7 days (Cole 2007).

References: Brown 2003; Cole 2007; George 2003; Koning 2004; Leyden 2003; Liu 2011; Oumeish 2000; Stevens 2005.

© 2013 Anti-infective Review Panel

Page 42 ‡ Common oral dosage ranges are provided unless otherwise stated. Consult the drug monograph for details on age and condition-specific dosing.

Modifying Circumstances	Probable Organism(s)	Antibiotic Choice(s)		Usual Dosage‡	Cost per Day

Cutaneous Infections: Uncomplicated [1, 2]

Modifying Circumstances	Probable Organism(s)	Antibiotic Choice(s)		Usual Dosage‡	Cost per Day
FOLLICULITIS[3] AND FURUNCLE[4] (BOIL)	S. aureus	FIRST LINE	Usually self limiting. Hot compresses and anti-septic cleanser may be beneficial. Systemic therapy not generally required.		
		SECOND LINE	Topical therapy in less severe / localized cases:		
			Mupirocin 2%[5] ung/cream	Apply sparingly TID	15 g ung: $5.33 15 g cr: $7.85
			Fusidic Acid 2%[5] ung/cream	Apply sparingly TID - QID. If covered with occlusive dressing, then daily or BID.	15 g: $8.74
CARBUNCLES[6] (MODERATE TO SEVERE)		FIRST LINE	Cephalexin	500 mg QID	$1.80
		SECOND LINE	Cloxacillin	500 mg QID	$1.40
			Clindamycin	300-450 mg QID	$1.77 - $2.66
		THIRD LINE	Erythromycin	1 g/day divided BID, TID or QID	$0.73
			Clarithromycin	250-500 mg BID	$0.82 - $1.65
			Azithromycin	500 mg daily on first day then 250 mg daily x 4 days	$1.57

1) Empiric coverage for methicillin resistant *S. aureus* (MRSA) should be considered **in areas where MRSA** is commonly isolated (>10-15% of *S. aureus*), in patients with prior antibiotic use or hospital admissions (over last 3-12 months) or recurrent furunculosis. TMP/SMX has activity against community-acquired MRSA, whereas cloxacillin, all cephalosporins and AM/CL do not. See treatment of CA-MRSA pages 51/52.

2) For dosing in CHILDREN, see impetigo on page 42.

3) Folliculitis is usually associated with an infected hair follicle. When assessing, try to determine whether it is infectious or not. Infectious folliculitis usually presents as bigger pustules (2-3 mm) vs pseudofolliculitis (1-2 mm), more inflammation (red halo and tenderness) and lesions tend to be clustered rather than scattered.

   Infectious folliculitis: Gram-ve folliculitis caused by Enterobacteriaceae may uncommonly develop in acne patients on long term antibiotics. When mild and limited, may respond to drying measures. Local compresses are beneficial. If no improvement or if disease is extensive, then topical antibacterial therapy should be used. Systemic therapy is generally not required unless the infection has progressed to the extent that it has become a carbuncle OR if scalp folliculitis is present.

   Pseudomonas folliculitis: Develops in individuals using hot-tubs contaminated with *Pseudomonas aeruginosa*. It has a predilection for the lower torso and the axillae. Typically self-limiting.

   Non-infectious folliculitis (or pseudofolliculitis): Inflammation of the hair follicle secondary to friction, irritation or occlusion. It is treated by removing the causative factor (i.e., friction or occlusion). Topical drying agents (e.g., aluminum chloride hexahydrate solution or a hydro-alcoholic solution) are beneficial.

4) Furuncles (boils) are abscesses that start in a hair follicle; for small boils hot compresses are usually sufficient, while for larger ones drainage is necessary. Culture if recurrent furuncles or abscesses (2 or more in 6 months). Antibiotics are generally unnecessary after incision and drainage of simple abscesses (Doung 2010; Schmitz 2010).

5) It has not been shown necessary to remove the crusts before application of fusidic acid or mupirocin.

6) Carbuncles are deeper and more extensive; incision and drainage is usually necessary. Consider systemic antibiotics if abscess ≥ 5 cm diameter, large and/or multiple abscesses, extensive surrounding cellulitis, located in central area of face, presence of constitutional symptoms or fever.

References: CREST 2005; Danziger 2002; Duong 2010; Pray 2000; Schmitz 2010; Stevens 2005; Stewart 2001; Stulberg 2002.

Modifying Circumstances	Probable Organism(s)	Antibiotic Choice(s)	Usual Dosage‡	Cost per Day

Cutaneous Infections: Complicated
(e.g., Perirectal Abscesses/Decubitus Ulcers) [1, 2]

Prevention is the best management for decubitus ulcers and abscesses. Local care may be adequate if there is no evidence of systemic infection or extensive ulceration. Incision/surgical drainage, debride and add antibiotics where necessary.

Modifying Circumstances	Probable Organism(s)	Antibiotic Choice(s)	Usual Dosage‡	Cost per Day
	Polymicrobial	**FIRST LINE** TMP/SMX [3] OR	1 - 2 DS tabs BID	$0.24 - $0.48
		Ciprofloxacin [4]	500 - 750 mg BID	$1.40 - $2.56
		± ONE of the following:		
		Metronidazole [5]	500 mg BID	$0.24
		Clindamycin [5]	300 - 450 mg QID	$1.77 - $2.66
		SECOND LINE Amoxicillin/Clavulanate [3, 5]	500 mg TID or 875 mg BID	$2.00
		Ceftriaxone IM/IV [6]	1 g q24h	$12.50
		± ONE of the following:		
		Metronidazole [5]	500 mg BID	$0.24
		Clindamycin [5]	300 - 450 mg QID	$1.77 - $2.66
		THIRD [7] LINE Cefazolin IV	1 - 2 g q8h	
		PLUS ONE of the following:		
		Metronidazole IV/PO	500 mg q12h	IV costs vary according to jurisdiction and/or contract pricing.
		Clindamycin IV/PO	PO: 300 - 450 mg QID IV: 600 mg q8h	
		PLUS ONE of the following:		
		Gentamicin IV [8]	4 - 7 mg/kg q24h	
		Tobramycin IV [8]	4 - 7 mg/kg q24h	
		Amikacin IV [8]	15 - 20 mg/kg q24h	

Continued ...

TMP/SMX = Trimethoprim / Sulfamethoxazole

‡ Common oral dosage ranges are provided unless otherwise stated. Consult the drug monograph for details on age and condition-specific dosing.

Cutaneous Infections: Complicated
(e.g., Perirectal Abscesses/Decubitus Ulcers)

1) Avoid topical antibiotic therapy and rule out osteomyelitis. Abscesses are often a significant problem requiring incision and drainage.

2) Empiric coverage for methicillin resistant *S. aureus* (MRSA) should be considered **in areas where MRSA** is commonly isolated (>10-15% of *S. aureus*) or in patients with prior antibiotic use or hospital admissions (over last 6-12 months). TMP/SMX is active against community-acquired MRSA, whereas cloxacillin, all cephalosporins and AM/CL do not. See treatment of CA-MRSA pages 51/52.

3) TMP/SMX or amoxicillin/clavulanate should not be used if *Pseudomonas* is present.

4) Consider using ciprofloxacin if *pseudomonas* is present.

5) If anaerobes are an issue, then clindamycin or metronidazole should be added. This will depend on the location (e.g., coccygeal ulcers, diabetic ulcers), spectrum of pathogens and severity of infection. Amoxicillin/clavulanate covers anaerobes and can be used alone.

6) Due to its long half-life, ceftriaxone may be used in emergency departments to avoid hospitalization in some cases.

7) Consideration can be given to using other agents including fluoroquinolones (levofloxacin, moxifloxacin), piperacillin-tazobactam, imipenem, meropenem or ertapenem in people with multiple drug allergies or as part of a multi-drug regimen.

8) For more information on aminoglycoside dosing, see page 109.

References: Barton 2006; Danziger 2002; Eron 2003; Livesley 2002; Muijsers 2002; Stevens 2005.

TMP/SMX = Trimethoprim / Sulfamethoxazole   © 2013 Anti-infective Review Panel

‡ Common oral dosage ranges are provided unless otherwise stated. Consult the drug monograph for details on age and condition-specific dosing. **Page 45**

Modifying Circumstances	Probable Organism(s)	Antibiotic Choice(s)		Usual Dosage‡	Cost per Day

Cellulitis – Uncomplicated: Mild [1, 2, 3]

Modifying Circumstances	Probable Organism(s)	Antibiotic Choice(s)		Usual Dosage‡	Cost per Day
ADULT AND CHILDREN	S. aureus Group A Strep.	FIRST LINE	Cephalexin	500 mg QID	$1.80
				Children: 50-100 mg/kg/day divided q6h	$0.06 - $0.13/kg
		SECOND LINE	Cloxacillin	500 mg QID	$1.40
				Children: 50 mg/kg/day divided q6h	$0.09/kg
			Clindamycin	300 mg QID	$1.77
				Children: 25 mg/kg/day	$0.19/kg
		THIRD LINE	Erythromycin (for adults)	1 g/day divided BID, TID or QID	$0.18
			Erythromycin estolate (for children)	**Children:** 30-40 mg/kg/day divided q12h	$0.03 - $0.04/kg
			Clarithromycin	250-500 mg BID	$0.82 - $1.65
				Children: 15 mg/kg/day divided q12h	$0.17/kg
			Azithromycin	500 mg daily on first day then 250 mg daily x 4 days	$1.57
				Children: 10 mg/kg/day on first day then 5 mg/kg x 4 days	$0.18/kg

1) If *Group A Strep.* is cultured then penicillin V or amoxicillin may be considered. If *S.aureus* is cultured cloxacillin can be used first line. If there is any doubt regarding the probable organism, cephalexin should be used.

2) Conditions that may masquerade as infectious cellulitis include: Vascular disorders (superficial and DVT); primary dermatological conditions (e.g., contact dermatitis, insect bites, drug reactions); rheumatic disorders (gouty arthritis); malignant disorders; foreign body reaction (e.g., metallic implant, silicone injections or mesh intolerance) (Fagalas 2005).

3) Empiric coverage for community acquired methicillin resistant *S. aureus* (CA-MRSA) should be considered **in areas where MRSA** is commonly isolated (>10-15% of *S. aureus*) or in patients with prior hospital admissions (over last 6-12 months) or where there is purulent drainage or exudate in the absence of a drainable abscess (Liu 2011).
TMP/SMX is active against community-acquired MRSA, whereas cloxacillin, all cephalosporins and AM/CL are not. See treatment of CA-MRSA pages 51/52.

References: CREST 2005; Danziger 2002; Falagas 2005; Liu 2011; Stevens 2005; Stewart 2001; Stulberg 2002; Swartz 2004; WATAG 2006.

Modifying Circumstances	Probable Organism(s)		Antibiotic Choice(s)	Usual Dosage‡	Cost per Day

Cellulitis – Uncomplicated: Severe (non-Facial) [1, 2]

Modifying Circumstances	Probable Organism(s)		Antibiotic Choice(s)	Usual Dosage‡	Cost per Day
ADULT AND CHILDREN	S. aureus Group A Strep. Group C Strep Group G Strep Group F Strep	FIRST LINE	Cefazolin IV	1 - 2 g q8h **Children;** 100 mg/kg/day divided q8h	$9.00 - $18.00 $0.30/kg
			±		
			Clindamycin PO	PO: 300 - 450 mg QID **Children:** 25 - 40 mg/kg/day divided QID	$1.77 - $2.66 $0.19 - $0.29/kg
			Alternative for Adults:		
			Cefazolin IV	2 g q24h	$6.00
			+		
			Probenecid PO	1 g once daily (Give 30 minutes prior to cefazolin)	$0.40
		SECOND LINE	Clindamycin IV [3]	600 mg q8h **Children:** 25 - 40 mg/kg/day divided q8h	$27.44 $0.38 - $0.61/kg
			Ceftriaxone IV/IM	1 g q24h **Children:** 75 mg/kg/day divided q12h-q24h (Maximum: 2 g/day)	$12.50 $1.60/kg
		THIRD LINE	Levofloxacin PO [3]	750 mg once daily x 5 days	$2.57 - $6.55
			Moxifloxacin PO [3]	400 mg once daily	$6.03

1) Conditions that may masquerade as infectious cellulitis include: Vascular disorders (superficial and DVT); primary dermatological conditions (e.g., contact dermatitis, insect bites, drug reactions); rheumatic disorders (gouty arthritis); malignant disorders; foreign body reaction (e.g., metallic implant, silicone injections or mesh intolerance) (Fagalas 2005).

2) Empiric coverage for community acquired methicillin resistant S. aureus (CA-MRSA) should be considered **in areas where MRSA** is commonly isolated (>10-15% of S. aureus) or in patients with prior hospital admissions (over last 6-12 months) or where there is purulent drainage or exudate in the absence of a drainable abscess (Liu 2011).
   TMP/SMX is active against community-acquired MRSA, whereas cloxacillin, all cephalosporins and AM/CL are not. See treatment of CA-MRSA pages 51/52.

3) Useful alternatives in cases of severe ß-lactam allergies (e.g., angioedema, bronchospasm, anaphylaxis, etc.).

References: CREST 2005; Danziger 2002; Falagas 2005; Grayson 2002; Liu 2011; Sibbald 2006; Stevens 2003; Stevens (IDSA) 2005; Stewart 2001; Stulberg 2002; Swartz 2004; WATAG 2006; Woo 2007, 2009.

TMP/SMX = Trimethoprim / Sulfamethoxazole

‡ Common oral dosage ranges are provided unless otherwise stated. Consult the drug monograph for details on age and condition-specific dosing.

Modifying Circumstances	Probable Organism(s)		Antibiotic Choice(s)	Usual Dosage‡	Cost per Day

Cellulitis – Special Considerations: Facial [1]

Modifying Circumstances	Probable Organism(s)		Antibiotic Choice(s)	Usual Dosage‡	Cost per Day
ADULT	Group A Strep. S. aureus	FIRST LINE	Cefazolin IV	1 - 2 g q8h	$9.00 - $18.00
			Ceftriaxone IM/IV [2]	1 g q24h	$12.50
		SECOND LINE	Clindamycin IV/PO	PO: 300 - 450 mg QID IV: 600 mg q8h	$1.77 - $2.66 $27.44
			Amoxicillin/Clavulanate [3]	500 mg TID or 875 mg BID	$2.00
		THIRD LINE	Vancomycin IV	1 g q12h	$31.00
CHILDREN	Group A Strep. S. aureus H. influenzae	FIRST LINE	Cefuroxime IV	100 - 150 mg/kg/day divided q8h	$2.15 - $3.23/kg
			Ceftriaxone IM/IV	75 mg/kg/day divided q12-q24h (Maximum: 2 g/day)	$1.60/kg
		SECOND LINE	Amoxicillin/Clavulanate [3]	40 mg/kg/day amoxicillin divided TID	$0.07/kg

Invasive Group A Strep [4, 5]: Necrotizing Fasciitis [6] (Adults Only)

Modifying Circumstances	Probable Organism(s)		Antibiotic Choice(s)	Usual Dosage‡	Cost per Day
	Group A Strep.	FIRST LINE	Clindamycin IV	600 mg q6h - q8h	$27.44 - $36.60
			PLUS ONE of the following:		
			Cefazolin IV	2 g q8h	$18.00
			OR		
			Penicillin G IV	12 - 24 million units/day divided q4-6h	$6.34 - $12.68
		SECOND LINE	Vancomycin IV	1 g q12h (15 mg/kg q12h: adjust dosing interval based on renal function)	$31.00

1) Consult infectious disease if MRSA suspected.
2) Suitable for outpatient settings where the patients can be reassessed q24h, or ideally, until parenteral therapy is no longer required. Use ceftriaxone if cellulitis is secondary to sinusitis. Cephalexin (500 mg QID x 7-10 days) can be used for outpatient management of mild facial cellulitis when *H. influenzae* has been ruled out.
3) Suitable as initial therapy ONLY in very mild cases of facial cellulitis.
4) Reportable to the Local Medical Officer of Health. Treat for a minimum of 10 days. Dosing regimens for polymicrobial infections or infections caused by organisms other than *Group A Strep* (e.g., mixed aerobic gram-negative bacilli and anaerobes) will differ. For prophylaxis of close household contacts, use cephalexin 250 mg PO QID x 10 days (alternatives: erythromycin or clindamycin).
5) IVIG (IV immunoglobulin) should be considered if toxic shock-like syndrome is present.
6) Surgery is an essential component of the management of necrotizing fasciitis.

References: Danziger 2002; Grayson 2002; Stevens 2003, 2005; Stewart 2001; Stulberg 2002; Swartz 2004.

‡ Common oral dosage ranges are provided unless otherwise stated. Consult the drug monograph for details on age and condition-specific dosing.

Modifying Circumstances	Probable Organism(s)		Antibiotic Choice(s)	Usual Dosage‡	Cost per Day

Cellulitis – Special Considerations: Diabetic Foot[1, 2]

Modifying Circumstances	Probable Organism(s)		Antibiotic Choice(s)	Usual Dosage‡	Cost per Day
MILD[3] TO MODERATE OR NON-LIMB THREATENING	S. aureus Group A Strep. Group B Strep. Enterococci P. aeruginosa[4] Mixed aerobic and anaerobic	FIRST LINE	[TMP/SMX[4]	1 - 2 DS tabs BID	$0.24 - $0.48
			OR		
			Cephalexin]	500 mg QID	$1.80
			PLUS		
			Metronidazole[1]	500 mg BID	$0.24
		SECOND LINE	Amoxicillin/Clavulanate[4, 5]	500 mg TID or 875 mg BID	$2.00
			OR		
			[TMP/SMX[4]	1 - 2 DS tabs BID	$0.24 - $0.48
			PLUS		
			Clindamycin[1]]	300 - 450 mg QID	$1.77 - $2.66
		THIRD[6] LINE	Cefazolin IV	1 - 2 g q8h	$9.00 - $18.00
			PLUS ONE of the following:		
			Metronidazole IV[1]	500 mg q12h	$3.78
			OR		
			Clindamycin IV[1]	600 mg q8h	$27.44

1) Deep cultures should be done in diabetic patients if the cellulitis is recurrent or associated with a long standing ulceration. Swabs of pus are useful, however surface swabs are not. **If anaerobes are an issue ("presence of necrotic tissue" or "foul smell"), clindamycin or metronidazole should be added. This will depend on the location, spectrum of pathogens and severity of infection.** Most non-limb threatening or mild infections are monomicrobial involving gram-positive bacteria only; therefore, it may not be necessary to cover for anaerobes; severe infections are usually polymicrobial, involving anaerobes.

2) Empiric coverage for methicillin resistant S. aureus (MRSA) should be considered in **areas where MRSA** is commonly isolated (>10-15% of S. aureus) or in patients with prior antibiotic use or hospital admissions over last 6-12 months. TMP/SMX is active against community-acquired MRSA, whereas cloxacillin, all cephalosporins and amoxicillin/clavulanate, are not. See treatment of CA-MRSA pages 51/52.

3) No evidence of systemic toxicity, deep tissue involvement, or spreading erythema. Non-limb threatening infections include superficial infections, < 2 cm cellulitis, no evidence of serious ischemia or systemic illness. Usually monomicrobial: S. aureus, Streptococci. Topical agents (including silver containing products) lack evidence for benefit and require further research before being recommended (Bergin 2006; McIntosh 2004). Cloxacillin 500 mg QID can be used if MSSA (methicillin sensitive S. aureus) is confirmed.

4) TMP/SMX or amoxicillin/clavulanate should not be used if Pseudomonas is present; use ciprofloxacin instead.

5) Amoxicillin/clavulanate covers anaerobes and can be used alone.

6) Diabetics have higher risk of decreased oral absorption due to gastric neuropathies, therefore IV antibiotics may be warranted initially or subsequent to poor response (at 2-4 days after initiation) to oral agents.

References: Bergin 2006; Calvet 2001; Crouzet 2011; Danziger 2002; Fong 1996; Frykburg 2006; Lipsky 2004; McIntosh 2004; Rose 2008; Sibbald 2006; Stevens (IDSA) 2005; University Health Network 2009; Woo 2009.

TMP/SMX = Trimethoprim / Sulfamethoxazole

‡ Common oral dosage ranges are provided unless otherwise stated. Consult the drug monograph for details on age and condition-specific dosing.

Modifying Circumstances	Probable Organism(s)	Antibiotic Choice(s)		Usual Dosage‡	Cost per Day

Cellulitis – Special Considerations: Diabetic Foot [1, 2, 3]

Modifying Circumstances	Probable Organism(s)	Antibiotic Choice(s)		Usual Dosage‡	Cost per Day
SEVERE [2] OR LIMB-THREATENING	S. aureus Group A Strep. Group B Strep. Enterococci P. aeruginosa [4] Mixed aerobic and anaerobic	FIRST LINE	Ceftriaxone IM/IV	1 - 2 g q24h	$12.50 - $24.14
			OR		
			Cefotaxime IV	1 - 2 g q8h	$27.60 - $55.20
			PLUS ONE of the following:		
			Metronidazole [1]	500 mg BID	$0.24
			Clindamycin [1]	300 - 450 mg QID	$1.77 - $2.66
		SECOND LINE	Ciprofloxacin PO/IV [4]	PO: 750 mg BID IV: 400 mg q12h	$2.56 $69.64
			PLUS		
			Clindamycin PO/IV [1]	PO: 300 - 450 mg QID IV: 600 mg q8h	$1.77 - $2.66 $27.44
		THIRD [5] LINE	Imipenem/Cilastatin IV	500 mg q6h	$97.52
			Piperacillin /Tazobactam IV	4.5 g / 0.5 g q8h	$63.66

1) Cultures should be taken. Consider admission to hospital. **If anaerobes are an issue ("presence of necrotic tissue" or "foul smell"), clindamycin or metronidazole should be added. This will depend on the location, spectrum of pathogens and severity of infection. Most non-limb threatening or mild infections are mono-microbial involving gram-positive bacteria only; therefore, it may not be necessary to cover for anaerobes; severe infections are usually polymicrobial, involving anaerobes. Duration of therapy 14-28 days if severe soft tissue infection. If bone involvement, consult osteomyelitis guideline; between 4 and 12 weeks generally required (Lipsky 2004).**

2) Severe as evidenced by systemic toxicity, deep tissue involvement or spreading erythema. Limb threatening infections include full thickness ulcer, > 2 cm cellulitis, serious ischemia. Usually polymicrobial. Note that topical agents (including silver containing products) lack evidence for benefit and require further research before use can be recommended (Bergin 2006; McIntosh 2003).

3) Empiric coverage for methicillin resistant S. aureus (MRSA) should be considered in **areas where MRSA** is commonly isolated (>10-15% of S. aureus) or in patients with prior antibiotic use or hospital admissions over the last 6-12 months. TMP/SMX is active against community-acquired MRSA, whereas cloxacillin, all cephalosporins and AM/CL are not. See treatment of CA-MRSA pages 51/52.

4) If it is known that *Pseudomonas* is present, specific agent is determined by susceptibilities (e.g., ciprofloxacin).

5) Consideration can be given to using other agents including meropenem, ertapenem or levofloxacin plus metronidazole, in patients with multiple drug allergies or as part of a multi-drug regimen.

References: Bergin 2006; Calvet 2001; Crouzet 2011; Danziger 2002; Fong 1996; Frykburg 2008; Lipsky 2004; McIntosh 2003; Sibbald 2006; University Health Network 2009; Woo 2009.

MRSA (Methicillin Resistant Staphylococcus Aureus)

MRSA is a potentially dangerous type of Staphylococcus bacteria that is resistant to certain antibiotics and may cause skin and other infections. MRSA-HA and CA are caused by different strains of MRSA and should both be treated based on susceptibility testing. See treatment table for CA-MRSA (Page 52).

- **CA-MRSA (community-associated):** Infections acquired by persons who have not been hospitalized within the last 12 months and do not have a history of surgery, dialysis, invasive device (catheter) or residence in a LTC facility. Usually manifests as skin infection, such as pimples and boils, and occurs in otherwise healthy, younger people. Generally appears as a bump or infected area on the skin (redness, swelling, pain, warm to the touch, full of pus or other drainage, fever). This is an emerging pathogen in Canada (Nichol 2009).

- **HA- MRSA (healthcare-associated):** Infections occur most frequently in hospital patients and those in non-hospital healthcare facilities (nursing homes, LTC and dialysis centres) who have weakened immune systems. Most common growth sites include: anterior nares, axilla, groin, perineum, rectum, skin ulcers, IV sites, indwelling catheters, tracheostomy and feeding tubes (Boyce 2008).

- **Colonization:** Occurs when MRSA is present in or on the body, but no clinical signs or symptoms of illness or infection are present. Colonized individuals may transmit MRSA, however decolonization is *not recommended in community settings* **because patients may become re-colonized when treatment stops and repeated decolonization for chronic carriers will contribute to the emergence of resistant organisms.** Prevention may be of only short duration, recolonization over time being the rule (Elliott 2009; Gorwitz 2006; Simor 2004). Only consider under exceptional circumstances (e.g., recurrent infections, transmission within a family) (PIDAC(a) 2011).

- **Infection:** MRSA infection may cause life-threatening infections and has been associated with institutional outbreaks. It causes significant morbidity and mortality, increased hospital length of stay and cost.

Suggestions for managing MRSA patients in office practice (Mattow 2009; PIDAC 2011(b), 2012):

- **Hand hygiene:** MRSA is almost always spread by direct physical contact and not through the air. Spread may also occur through indirect contact by touching objects such as towels, sheets, wound dressings and clothes contaminated by the infected skin of a person with MRSA. Ensure appropriate sterilization of all patient care equipment with hospital grade disinfectant following visit.
- When dealing with an open wound: gloves, mask, gown, contact isolation, barrier precautions.
- Book MRSA patients at the end of the clinic day and educate office staff about reducing MRSA spread.
- Judicious use of antibiotics is one of the most effective ways of preventing emergence of MRSA. De-colonization is not generally warranted.

Patient Education:

1. **Precautions when Patient with MRSA is at Home**

   Outside of healthcare settings healthy people are at low risk of getting infected. Precautions include:
   - Caregivers should wash their hands with soap and water after physical contact with the infected or colonized person and before leaving the home.
   - Towels used for drying hands after contact should be used only once; paper towels recommended.
   - Avoid sharing personal items, such as towels and razors.
   - Disposable gloves should be worn if contact with body fluids is expected and hands washed following their removal.
   - Linens should be changed and washed if they are soiled and on a routine basis.
   - The patient's environment should be cleaned routinely and when soiled with body fluids.
   - Notify doctors and other healthcare personnel who provide care for the patient that the patient is colonized or infected with a multidrug-resistant organism.

2. **Precautions when Patient with MRSA is in a Facility**
   - Healthy people are at low risk of getting infected with MRSA.
   - Casual contact such as kissing, hugging and touching is acceptable.
   - Visitors should wash their hands before leaving an infected person's room.
   - Disposable gloves should be worn if contact with body fluids is expected.
   - If excessive contact with body fluids is expected, gowns should also be worn.
   - It is also acceptable for infants and children to have casual contact with these patients.

References: Barton 2006; Beam 2006; Boyce 2008; Conly 2002; Elliott 2009; Gorwitz 2006; Johnston 2008; Lui 2011; Mattow 2009; Mulvey 2005; Nathwani 2008; Nichol 2009; Nicolle 2006; PIDAC 2011(a, b), 2012; Simor 2004.

Modifying Circumstances	Probable Organism(s)	Antibiotic Choice(s)		Usual Dosage‡	Cost per Day

Community-acquired MRSA -Normal Host [1, 2, 3, 4]

Modifying Circumstances	Probable Organism(s)	Antibiotic Choice(s)		Usual Dosage‡	Cost per Day
MINOR SKIN LESIONS		Localized disease (infected scratches, furuncles, small abscesses) can usually be managed with topical therapy (mupirocin and/or topical antiseptics), elevation, local incision and drainage. Reassess if no improvement or if condition worsens.			
		Does not apply to immunocompromised host or neonates.			
ADULT & CHILDREN **MODERATE** (cellulitis, abscesses, minimal systemic features)	*S. aureus*	**FIRST LINE**	**TMP/SMX** [5]	2 tabs BID-QID or 1 DS tab BID-QID **Children:** 8-12 mg/kg/day TMP component divided q12h	$0.08 - $0.24 $0.02 - $0.03/kg
			Doxycycline	100 mg BID **(Children > 8 years of age)**	$1.17
			Clindamycin	150-450 mg QID **Children:** 25-30 mg/kg/day divided q6-8h	$0.89 - $2.66 $0.19 - $0.20/kg
SEVERE (extensive cellulitis, multiple abscesses with systemic features)		**FIRST LINE**	**Vancomycin IV**	1 g q12h **Children:** 10 mg/kg q6h	$31.00
			Linezolid	400-600 mg q12h **Children ≤ 11y:** 20 mg/kg q12h **Children < 5y:** 10 mg/kg q8h	600 mg: $70.64 susp. 2 mg/mL: $95.50

1) **Prevention:** Judicious use of antibiotics; hand hygiene; not sharing personal care items (e.g., towels, soap); early recognition, containment and management of infections if they do occur.

2) **CA-MRSA** has a predilection to skin and soft tissue infections, producing cellulitis and abscesses. It may cause necrotizing community acquired pneumonia, septic shock, or bone and joint infections. **Screening for nasopharyngeal carriage or carriage at other sites is not recommended and decolonization therapy is generally discouraged due to likelihood of producing even more resistant strains** (Mulvey 2005).

3) **When to suspect CA-MRSA:** Any patient who presents with a skin or soft tissue infection in a community where > 10-15% of all *S. aureus* isolates are MRSA; patients from high-risk groups (athlete contact sports, institutionalized, incarcerated, homeless, parenteral drug users, HIV, malnutrition); any patient who has not responded to treatment with a ß-lactam antibiotic; prior antimicrobial therapy (especially broad spectrum) in last 6 months; invasive procedures/devices (e.g., dialysis, indwelling catheter); advanced age, young adults, children < 2 years.

4) **Management:** Culture any lesion that is potentially caused by MRSA. Even minor lesions should be cultured if a patient with multiple skin lesions is a member of a high-risk group or if ß-lactam therapy has failed. **Limit antimicrobial therapy where possible.** Note that even in areas that are endemic for CA-MRSA, ß-lactams (cephalexin) are still considered appropriate first line empiric therapy for soft skin and tissue infections (Elliott 2009). Cephalexin 500 mg QID can be used in conjunction with TMP/SMX and doxycycline. The current rate of CA-MRSA susceptibility to clindamycin is approximately 89% vs 100% for TMP/SMX (CARA 2009).

5) **Sulfamethoxazole-trimethoprim (TMP/SMX)** was originally introduced as a treatment for cystitis at an adult dose of 2 regular tablets (1 DS tablet) BID; the aim was to achieve therapeutic levels in the urine, not the blood or tissues. When pneumocystis carinii pneumonia (PCP) became common with the onset of HIV-AIDS, the TMP/SMX dose for that indication was quadrupled to 2 DS tablets QID for three weeks. For treating mild to moderate MRSA infections of the skin and soft tissues, a higher dose is required in order to achieve effective tissue concentrations. Although there is no data from randomized studies, a middle-ground adult dose of 1 DS tablet (2 regular tablets) QID would appear to be prudent and is being used successfully in clinical practice; this is half the dose used for PCP. For children with MRSA skin and soft-tissue infections, the otitis-media dose could be doubled (Pennie 2010).

References: Barton 2006; Boyce 2005, 2008; CARA 2009; Conly 2002; Duong 2010; Elliott 2009; File 2007; Gilbert 2006; Gorwitz 2006; Irvine 2012; Johnston 2008; Klevens 2007; Liu 2011; Moore 2012; Mulvey 2005; Nathwani 2008; Nichol 2009; Nicolle 2005, 2006; Pennie 2010; Popovich 2008; Robinson 2011; Schmitz 2010; Siegel 2007; Simor 2004; Skiest 2007; TOP 2010.

© 2013 Anti-infective Review Panel   TMP/SMX = Trimethoprim / Sulfamethoxazole

Page 52   ‡ Common oral dosage ranges are provided unless otherwise stated. Consult the drug monograph for details on age and condition-specific dosing.

Modifying Circumstances	Probable Organism(s)	Antibiotic Choice(s)		Usual Dosage‡	Cost per Day

Bites: Cat, Dog, Wild Animal and Human [1, 2, 3]

Modifying Circumstances	Probable Organism(s)	Antibiotic Choice(s)		Usual Dosage‡	Cost per Day
MILD INFECTION	P. multiocida [4] S. aureus Viridans Strep. Bacteroides Fusobacter C. canimorsus Anaerobic streptococci Eikenella corrodens	FIRST LINE	Amoxicillin/Clavulanate	500 mg TID or 875 mg BID	$2.00
				Children: 40 mg/kg/day amoxicillin divided q8h	$0.07/kg
		SECOND LINE	Doxycycline [5]	100 mg BID first day then 100 mg once daily	$0.59
				Children: 2 - 4 mg/kg/day q12h on first day then half dose q24h	$0.34 - $0.68/kg
			Ceftriaxone IM/IV	1 - 2g q24h	$12.50 - $24.14
				Children: 50 - 100 mg/kg/day q24h	$0.85 - $1.70/kg
MODERATE TO SEVERE INFECTION		FIRST LINE	Ceftriaxone IM/IV [6]	1 - 2g q24h	$12.50 - $24.14
			±	**Children:** 50 - 100 mg/kg/day q24h	$0.85 - $1.70/kg
			Metronidazole [7]	500 mg BID	$0.24
		SECOND LINE	Ticarcillin/Clavulanate IV [8]	3.1g q4-6h	$40.40 - $60.60
				Children: 200 - 300 mg/kg/day divided q4-6h	$0.62 - $0.93/kg
			Piperacillin/Tazobactam IV [8]	3 g/0.375 g q6h	$62.00
				Children: 200 - 300 mg/kg/day divided q8h	$1.09 - $1.64/kg
		If allergic to Beta-lactam antibiotics			
			[TMP/SMX PO/IV	4 - 5 mg/kg/day divided q6-12h	PO: $0.01/kg 5 mL vial: $5.75
			OR		
			Ciprofloxacin]	500 mg BID	$1.40
			±		
			Metronidazole [7]	500 mg BID	$0.24
			OR		
			Clindamycin	300 - 450 mg QID	$1.77 - $2.66

TMP/SMX = Trimethoprim / Sulfamethoxazole   © 2013 Anti-infective Review Panel

‡ Common oral dosage ranges are provided unless otherwise stated. Consult the drug monograph for details on age and condition-specific dosing.   **Page 53**

Bites: Cat, Dog, Wild Animal and Human

1) All wounds should be thoroughly cleaned, irrigated and debrided. Ensure tetanus prophylaxis is up to date. Duration of treatment is usually 7 to 14 days, or longer if there is bone or joint involvement.

2) Refer to the Canadian Immunization Guide for management of rabies. Report to local public health office if potentially exposed to rabies (e.g., wild or domestic animal bite).

3) Prophylaxis with antibiotics is controversial, but is almost always recommended for high-risk wounds, such as deep punctures, wounds to the face or upper limbs, other joints or cartilaginous structures, those inflicted through unprovoked attacks or wild animals (Medeiros 2001; Rittner 2005; Foreshew 2006; Can Paed Soc 2008). Twenty-eight percent to 80% of cat and 3% to 28% of dog bites result in infection; therefore, prophylaxis against feline bites may be given more consideration (Rittner 2005; Singer 2008).

   Human-Pediatric: Where biting has occurred between children, consider prophylactic antibiotics if there is moderate to severe tissue damage, deep puncture wounds or bites to the face, hand, foot or genitals that are more than simple superficial abrasion. Usual prophylactic course of therapy is 3 to 5 days (NHS 2008; PIER 2008). If a child known to be a Hepatitis B (HBV) carrier bites and breaks the skin of a non-immune child, Hepatitis B immunoglobulin 0.06 ml/kg IM and HBV vaccine should be administered to the bitten child. If the biter is non-immune and bites a HBV carrier, HBV vaccine should be given to the biter. Where the status of the biter or victim is unknown, low risk does not warrant HBV testing (Paed Child Health 2008).

   Human-Adult: Assess for risks of blood borne pathogen transmission and treat appropriately (NHS 2008).

4) *P. multocida* is resistant to erythromycin, clindamycin, 1st generation cephalosporins and cloxacillin.

5) In children under 9 years of age, the use of tetracyclines is not generally recommended.

6) **Outpatient treatment of moderate to severe bites has been successful with 1 g ceftriaxone IV or IM x 2-4 days, followed by oral antibiotics, usually amoxicillin 500 mg TID.** The IM protocol can be easily administered in-office, in emergency departments, or through home care programs in order to avoid hospitalization (Pennie 2004).

7) Metronidazole is more important for human bites since anaerobic coverage is required.

8) *Eikenella corrodens* is resistant to ticarcillin and piperacillin, hence, these agents may not be appropriate in human bites.

References: Can Paed Soc 2008; Foreshew 2006; Kravetz 2008; Medeiros 2001; Morgan 2007; NHS 2008; Paed Child Health 2008; Pennie 2004; PIER 2008; Rittner 2005; Singer 2008; Stevens 2005; Swartz 2004.

Modifying Circumstances	Probable Organism(s)		Antibiotic Choice(s)	Usual Dosage‡	Cost per Day

Lyme Disease [1, 2, 3, 4]

Modifying Circumstances	Probable Organism(s)		Antibiotic Choice(s)	Usual Dosage‡	Cost per Day
ADULTS	B. burgdorferi	FIRST LINE	Amoxicillin	500 mg TID	$1.03
			Doxycycline [3, 5]	100 mg BID	$1.17
		SECOND LINE	Cefuroxime-AX	500 mg BID	$2.87
		THIRD LINE [6]	Ceftriaxone IV	2 g q24h	$24.14
			Cefotaxime IV	2 g q8h	$55.20
			Penicillin G IV	3 - 4 million units q4h	$9.51 - $12.68
CHILDREN	B. burgdorferi	FIRST LINE	Amoxicillin	50 mg/kg/day divided q8h	$0.03/kg
		SECOND LINE	Cefuroxime-AX	30 mg/kg/day divided q12h	$0.66/kg
			Doxycycline [3, 5]	2 - 4 mg/kg/day divided q12h	$0.01 - $0.02/kg
		THIRD LINE [6]	Ceftriaxone IV	75 - 100 mg/kg/day divided q24h	$1.19 - $1.58/kg
			Cefotaxime IV	100 - 180 mg/kg/day divided q6-8h	$0.45 - $0.60/kg
			Penicillin G IV	200,000 - 400,000 U/kg/day divided q4h	$1.06 - $2.11/kg

1) Adapted from IDSA Practice Guidelines for the Treatment of Lyme Disease (Wormser 2006).

2) Reportable to Local Medical Officer of Health. Humans can contract Lyme disease without visiting endemic areas; it should not be excluded from differential diagnosis based on geographic location unless the location is sufficiently northern to preclude migratory birds from dropping their tics in the area (PHAC 2008). Expansion of the geographic range of the tic vector in Canada is leading to increasing numbers of endemic areas for Lyme disease (Ogden 2009).

3) Usual duration of therapy is 14-21 days. In patients with early localized disease, 10 days of doxycycline treatment has proven effective for erythema migrans/early localized stage of disease and where there is disseminated cardiac involvement (Wormser 2006). For patients who have had improvement during or after a course of oral antibiotics but who have persistent or recurrent joint swelling, a second four week course of oral antibiotics is recommended (Halperin 2009). Prolonged courses of antibiotics provide no additional benefits and should be discouraged (Fallon 2008; Klempner 2001; Krupp 2003; Sider 2012; Wormser 2007).

4) Lyme disease must be considered whenever neurologic disease occurs in association with significant constitutional or extraneural features. Neurologic involvement occurs in 10-40% of symptomatic infections and occurs at all stages of infection. Patients with early local disease may experience mild headache, stiff neck, fatigue and myalgias. The dissemination stage is associated with certain neurologic syndromes that tend to improve spontaneously after several weeks to months without treatment. Cases have been documented in all regions of Ontario. Serologic testing to diagnose Lyme disease is a source of controversy since specific antibodies may not be detectable until four to six weeks after the initial infection. One should not complete the test in the absence of good epidemiological evidence of infection (PHAC 2008).

5) The use of tetracyclines in children under 9 years of age and pregnant women is not generally recommended.

6) Parenteral therapy (generally 14-28 days) should be considered in patients with acute neurological disease (meningitis or radiculopathy), 3rd degree heart block, CNS or peripheral nervous system disease in late Lyme disease, and in cases of recurrent arthritis after oral regimens of 1-2 months have been used.

References: Baker 2010; CPHLN 2007; Fallon 2008; Halperin 2007, 2009; Hengge 2003; Klempner 2001; Krupp 2003; Lantos 2010; Ogden 2009; PHAC 2008; Robinson 2011; Sider 2012; Wormser 2006, 2007.

© 2013 Anti-infective Review Panel

Common oral dosage ranges are provided unless otherwise stated. Consult the drug monograph for details on age and condition-specific dosing. **Page 55**

Modifying Circumstances	Probable Organism(s)	Antibiotic Choice(s)	Usual Dosage‡	Cost per Day

Herpes Simplex Virus – Mucocutaneous [1]
(Normal Host)

Modifying Circumstances	Probable Organism(s)	Antibiotic Choice(s)	Usual Dosage‡	Cost per Day
COLD SORES First or occasional episodes	Herpes Simplex type 1 or 2	**No therapy recommended**		
Severe, recurrent episodes (> 3/year) [2]	Herpes Simplex type 1 or 2	**Famciclovir** [3] **Valacyclovir** [3]	500 mg BID x 7 days 2 g BID x 1 day	$3.38 $6.79
LOCALIZED LESIONS		**No treatment unless direct dissemination, then use acyclovir**		
LOCALIZED BUT CHRONIC (PERI-ANAL)		**See Genital Herpes in Genitourinary section**		
GINGIVAL STOMATITIS [4]		**No definitive recommendations available**		

(Immunocompromised Host)

		No general recommendations for immunocompromised hosts. Individualize therapy and consult specialist as needed.		

1) Topical treatment (e.g., acyclovir, docosanol) has not shown definitive efficacy or comparative superiority to other treatments. It must be commenced during the prodromal stage.

2) For continuous suppression in an adult or child with > 6 recurrences per year acyclovir 400 mg BID (children: acyclovir 10 mg/kg/dose BID to maximum 400 mg) has been used (Jones 2004).

3) Valacyclovir has shown prevention of lesion progression and shortening of symptoms by 1 day if self initiated by patient an average of 2 hours after the earliest symptom. Fluocinonide 0.05% topical cream (e.g., Lidex, Lyderm, etc.) q8h x 5 days in combination with valacyclovir has shown improvement over valacyclovir monotherapy. Famciclovir has shown shortening of symptoms by 2 days. These medications should be commenced during the prodromal stage of presentation.

4) Gingival Stomatitis: HSV initial infection peaks in children between 9 months and 3 years of age. Lesions are usually noted on the mucosa and are self-limiting. Acyclovir oral 15 mg/kg to a maximum of 200 mg five times daily for 7 days has been found to reduce symptoms if started within 72 hours (Jones 2004; Nasser 2008).

References: Aoki 2006; Brady 2004; CAN STI 2008; CDC 2006; CKS 2007; Jones 2004; Laiskonis 2002; Nasser 2008; Prodigy 2003; Raborn 2004; Spruance 2002, 2003; Straten 2001.

© 2013 Anti-infective Review Panel

Page 56   ‡ Common oral dosage ranges are provided unless otherwise stated. Consult the drug monograph for details on age and condition-specific dosing.

Modifying Circumstances	Probable Organism(s)		Antibiotic Choice(s)	Usual Dosage‡	Cost per Day

Herpes Simplex Virus – Keratitis or Keratoconjunctivitis [1,2]

Modifying Circumstances	Probable Organism(s)		Antibiotic Choice(s)	Usual Dosage‡	Cost per Day
ADULTS AND CHILDREN	Herpes Simplex type 1 or 2	*FIRST LINE*	**Trifluridine [3] ophthalmic solution**	Instill 1 drop onto cornea q2h while awake (Maximum daily dose: 9 drops). Continue until lesion re-epithelialized then 1 drop q4h (Maximum daily dose: 5 drops) for 7 days.	7.5 mL: $22.79

1) Presentation: Red, irritated, watery eye often accompanied by multiple vesicles on eyelid but may also involve face. Eyelid edema and ulcers may be present; may involve cornea. Consult an ophthalmologist. Also, for the prevention of recurrent herpes simplex virus (HSV) eye disease, consultation with an ophthalmologist is recommended.

2) Do not use any topical-steroid-containing preparation alone. In certain cases, concurrent use of steroids with antivirals may be necessary to treat progressive inflammation as in uveitis or stromal keratitis (Wutzler 1997). Corticosteroids can cause an ocular herpetic ulcer to degrade into an extensive amoeboid ulcer resulting in potential scarring and visual loss.

3) If there are no signs of improvement after 7 days of full therapy or complete re-epithelialization has not occurred after 14 days of full therapy, other forms of therapy should be considered. Administration of a full dosage regimen for periods exceeding 21 days should be avoided because of potential ocular toxicity.

References: Brady 2004; CAN STI 2008; CDC 2006; Evans 2011; Jones 2004; Lairson 2003; Laiskonis 2002; Prodigy 2003; Wilhelmus 2010.

© 2013 Anti-infective Review Panel

‡ Common oral dosage ranges are provided unless otherwise stated. Consult the drug monograph for details on age and condition-specific dosing. **Page 57**

Varicella Zoster Virus – Shingles [1, 2, 3, 4]
(Normal Host)

ADULT		Initiate within 72 hours of rash onset [5]		
	FIRST LINE	Famciclovir	500 mg TID for 7 days	$5.07
		Valacyclovir	1 g TID for 7 days	$5.09
	SECOND LINE	Acyclovir	800 mg 5 times daily for 7 days	$6.34
		Acyclovir IV	10 mg/kg/dose q8h	500 mg vial: $66.15

(Immunocompromised Host) [6]

		Initiate within 72 hours of rash onset [5]		
	FIRST LINE	Acyclovir IV	10 mg/kg/dose q8h for 7-14 days	500 mg vial: $66.15
			Children: IV: < 1 yr: 10 mg/kg/dose q8h for 7-14 days IV: ≥ 1 yr: 500 mg/m^2/dose q8h for 7-14 days	
			PO (following IV): 20 mg/kg/dose QID	PO: $0.23/kg

1) Topical antivirals are not recommended. Role of steroids is controversial; a recent review indicated no benefit for post-herpetic neuralgia with steroids, however acute pain may be improved with 7-14 day treatment with systemic corticosteroids (He 2008). Risks may outweigh benefits. Consult with a specialist before initiating steroid treatment in acute varicella zoster.

2) Immunocompetent children less than 12 years of age with shingles usually do not require treatment with antivirals unless the disease shows signs of dissemination (Klassen 2004; Marin 2007). Consider treatment in children > 11 years of age; chronic cutaneous or pulmonary disorders; chronic steroid or salicylate therapy.

3) Consider seeking specialist advice in cases of shingles in pregnancy.

4) Varcella zoster vaccine (Zostavax-0.65 mL single dose s.c. injection) is indicated for the prevention of shingles in immunocompetent patients ≥ 60 years old and may be used in persons 50-59 years of age (Li 2012; NACI 2010). Efficacy is highest in patients 60-69 years old and decreases with increasing age. Post-vaccination the efficacy of the vaccine decreases yearly, losing statistical significance after 3 years for post-herpetic neuralgia (PHN) and after 6 years for shingles (Schmader 2012). NNT: for every 364 patients vaccinated, 6 cases of shingles & 1 case of PHN is prevented over 3 years (Brisson 2008). Following a prior episode of herpes zoster, consider delaying vaccination ≥ 1 year to take advantage of this natural immunity (Zang 2012).

5) Initiation of antivirals may be considered for up to one week after rash onset if there is a high risk of severe shingles or complications (severe pain, old age or continued vesicle emergence). Use of antivirals is strongly advocated in patients ≥ 50 years of age or in patients with one of: moderate or severe pain, moderate or severe rash or non-truncal involvement.

6) In severe zoster infections (e.g., multiple dermatomes, disseminated or trigeminal nerve involvement), IV acyclovir should be used. In mildly to moderately immunocompromised hosts with localized shingles or after infection control is established, oral famciclovir or valacyclovir is an acceptable alternative to IV therapy, or as step-down therapy from IV therapy (Dworkin 2007; Kempf 2007). HIV patients require treatment until all lesions have healed (longer than the standard 7-14 day course).

References: Brisson 2008; CADTH 2006; CDC 2012; Dworkin 2007; Fekete 2005; Harpaz 2008; He 2008; Kempf 2007; Kimberlin 2007; Klassen 2004; Li 2012; Marin 2007; NACI 2010; Oxman 2005; Schmader 2012; Shafran 2004; Shapiro 2011; Wareham 2007.

Modifying Circumstances	Probable Organism(s)	Antibiotic Choice(s)		Usual Dosage‡	Cost per Day

Varicella Zoster Virus – Shingles (continued)
(V1 Zoster or Zoster Ophthalmicus) [1, 2]

Modifying Circumstances		Antibiotic Choice(s)		Usual Dosage‡	Cost per Day
NON-OPHTHALMIC OR OPHTHALMIC	*ORAL*	Famciclovir		500 mg TID x 7-10 days **Children:** not indicated	$5.07
		Valacyclovir		1 g TID x 7-10 days **Children:** not indicated	$5.09
	IV	Acyclovir		10 mg/kg q8h or 30 mg/kg/day for a minimum of 5 days **Children:** IV: $\geq$ 1 year: 500 mg/m^2 q8h PO: (following IV): 20 mg/kg/dose QID	500 mg vial: $66.15 PO: $0.23/kg

1) Consult an ophthalmologist if there is eye or nasociliary involvement. A topical antibiotic ophthalmic ointment (possibly with steroid) twice daily may be warranted to protect the ocular surface and decrease inflammation (Dworkin 2007).

2) Clinical benefits are more evident if therapy is initiated within 48 hours of onset of symptoms, where the incidence of uveitis and keratitis were reduced compared to placebo (Snoeck 1999).

References: AOA 2002; Dworkin 2007; Gnann 2002; Gross 2003; Shafran 2004; Snoeck 2004.

‡ Common oral dosage ranges are provided unless otherwise stated. Consult the drug monograph for details on age and condition-specific dosing.

Modifying Circumstances	Probable Organism(s)		Antibiotic Choice(s)	Usual Dosage‡	Cost per Day

Chicken Pox – Treatment and Post-exposure Prevention [1,2]
(Normal Host)

			ADULTS [1]		
TREATMENT	Varicella-zoster virus (VZV)	FIRST LINE	If treatment is to have any benefit, initiate within 24 hours of onset of rash		
			Famciclovir	500 mg TID	$5.07
			Valacyclovir	1 g TID	$5.09
		SECOND LINE	Acyclovir	20 mg/kg/dose QID (Maximum: 800 mg/dose QID)	800 mg: $1.27
PREVENTION			Chickenpox vaccine [2]	Within 72 hours of exposure	

			DURING PREGNANCY [3]		
TREATMENT			Acyclovir IV	10 mg/kg/dose q8h	500 mg: $66.15
			Acyclovir PO	20 mg/kg/dose QID (Maximum: 800 mg/dose QID)	800 mg: $1.27
PREVENTION			VariZIG IM [3]	125 units (1 vial)/10 kg (Maximum: 625 units) (optimal dose for adults is uncertain)	

			CHILDREN		
TREATMENT			Not recommended routinely [4]		
PREVENTION			Chickenpox vaccine [2]	Within 72 hours of exposure	

			NEONATES		
TREATMENT			Acyclovir IV	10 mg/kg/dose q8h	500 mg: $66.15
PREVENTION			VariZIG IM [5]	125 units (1 vial)/10 kg (Maximum: 625 units)	

(Immunocompromised Host) [6]

			ADULTS AND CHILDREN		
TREATMENT			Acyclovir IV	10 mg/kg/dose q8h (**Children:** 500 mg/m^2 q8h)	500 mg: $66.15
PREVENTION			VariZIG and chickenpox vaccine may be considered for post-exposure prevention in immunocompromised adults and children who have NOT had chickenpox or the vaccine previously.		

Continued ...

Chicken Pox – Treatment and Post-exposure Prevention
(Normal Host)

1) Reportable to the Local Medical Officer of Health. There is no good quality evidence to support using antiviral therapy in otherwise healthy adults. Clinical benefit may consist of reduction in lesion number and time to full crusting, at best. Benefit increases in immunocompromised patients and those with concomitant skin or pulmonary conditions. **Duration of therapy:** 5-7 days in general; in cases where infection is associated with pneumonia or visceral involvement or in immunocompromised patients longer, duration is warranted. In cases where there is evidence or suspicion of chickenpox pneumonitis, encephalitis or hepatitis, IV acyclovir therapy may be considered regardless of time of onset of symptoms.

2) Chickenpox vaccine is now included as a routine immunization in paediatrics by Health Canada; pre-vaccine cohorts who have not had chickenpox may be at increased risk for shingles outbreaks. Post-exposure prophylaxis with chickenpox vaccine is effective in preventing or attenuating disease in previously healthy persons if the vaccine can be carried out within 3-5 days of exposure. There is some evidence to support its use in children under 16 years of age (NNT to prevent 1 case if given within 5 days of exposure = 2). Ideally administration should occur within the first 72h of exposure, but can be considered for up to 5 days post-exposure. The varicella vaccine is contraindicated in pregnant women, however susceptible pregnant women should be given the vaccine after delivery as long as 5 months have passed since varicella zoster immune globulin administration.

3) **Pregnant women:** Due to greater risk of severe illness and death from chickenpox, varicella zoster immune globulin should be considered in pregnant women who are **non-immune** (have never had varicella disease, shingles or varicella vaccine), **varicella-zoster immunoglobulin G (IgG) antibody negative** and who have had **significant exposure** (household contact, face-to-face contact with case for >15 minutes or contact indoors with a case for > 1 hour) within the last 96 hours. Where possible, blood should be obtained to determine varicella zoster antibody status since negative histories from adults about prior chickenpox are not very reliable (70-90% of those with a negative history are immune). A positive history is very reliable in indicating immunity. If seronegative, administer VariZIG up to 10 days post-exposure (Alberta Health and Wellness 2008; NACI 2006; NHS-CKS 2007; RCOG 2007).

   Guidelines differ on antiviral implementation criteria in pregnancy with some advocating for use of acyclovir or valacyclovir within 24h of rash onset at any gestational age and others suggesting only after 20 weeks of gestation. There is a small risk of fetal varicella syndrome and a greater risk of the mother experiencing serious complications of varicella (e.g., fulminating varicella pneumonia) during the 2nd and early 3rd trimester (NHS-CKS 2009; RCOG 2007).

4) Oral acyclovir cannot be recommended routinely for the treatment of uncomplicated chickenpox in otherwise healthy children (Klassen 2005). In children at increased risk of severe chickenpox due to concurrent cutaneous or pulmonary disorders, in an immunocompromised state (on high dose steroids or taking salicylates chronically) or if >13 years of age, antiviral treatment should be considered if it can be initiated within 72h of rash onset with acyclovir 10-20 mg/kg QID for 5 to 7 days.

5) Infants born to mothers who develop chickenpox during the period 5 days before to 2 days after delivery should receive VariZIG as soon as possible after delivery in order to reduce the risk of severe or fatal chickenpox. If this fails and chickenpox develops, the infant should be hospitalized and treated with acyclovir IV 30 mg/kg/day, divided into 3 daily doses for 7 days. Exposed infants of < 28 weeks' gestational age should receive VariZIG regardless of maternal immune status. Exposed infants 29-37 weeks' gestational age should receive VariZIG if the mother was not immune (NACI 2006).

6) Susceptible immunocompromised patients with significant exposure should be given a prescription for acyclovir and counseled regarding the fact that the onset of chickenpox is usually a fever and a feeling of unwellness before the rash. The prescription should be filled if any febrile illness occurs, or if any rash appears. Oral antivirals may be considered (see doses in normal host section) in non-severe cases.

References: Alberta Health and Wellness 2012; Allen 2006; Can Paed Soc 2005; Klassen 2005; Macartney 2008; Marin 2007; NACI 2006 (a,b); NHS-CKS 2009; RCOG 2007; SOGC 2012.

Genitourinary Infections

Acute Urinary Tract Infection (UTI) – *Clinical Decision Aid* [1, 2]

In general practice, empirical treatment of acute cystitis may result in up to 40% of women with urinary symptoms receiving antibiotics unnecessarily for negative urine culture results (McIsaac 2002). The following is a tool provided to assist in the treatment (NOT diagnosis) of patients presenting with acute cystitis.

Step 1

If AFTER completing your clinical assessment you conclude the patient likely has uncomplicated acute cystitis, determine the number of the following criteria that are present:

Criteria	Points
• Burning or pain on urination	1
• Presence of leukocytes (more than a trace amount)	1
• Presence of nitrites (any positive, including trace amount)	1

Step 2

SUGGESTED management according to total number of criteria (and if your clinical judgement does not identify additional factors that suggest the approach should be modified)

Total Score	Risk of Positive Urine Culture	Suggested Management
0 - 1	26-38 %	• Perform urine culture before deciding about the need for antibiotics. Treat with empiric therapy if symptoms are severe.
2 - 3	> 70 %	• Start empirical antimicrobial therapy without waiting for urine cultures owing to the high likelihood of infection.

1) Adapted from McIsaac 2007. This is a validated score for community-based family practice.
2) Appropriate to start empiric therapy if patient is uncomfortable and feels symptoms are severe or if patient is unwilling to wait for culture results.

Recurrent vs Reinfection vs Relapse?

Recurrent:	• Two uncomplicated UTIs within 6 months OR
	• Three or more positive urine cultures in the prior 12 months

Reinfection:
- Occurs after 2 weeks of completing antimicrobial therapy
- Caused by a different organism
- Most common
- Follows ascension of microorganisms from the periurethral area into the bladder

Relapse:
- Generally occurs within 2 weeks of completing antimicrobial treatment
- Caused by the original organism
- Bacteriuria often persists during therapy or reoccurs after 1-2 weeks of finishing antimicrobial therapy
- Occurs in a minority of women (5-10%)

> **Always consider local antimicrobial susceptibilities and resistance rates in addition to a patient's recent antimicrobial use.**

Modifying Circumstances	Probable Organism(s)		Antibiotic Choice(s)	Usual Dosage‡	Cost per Day

Acute Urinary Tract Infection – Female: Uncomplicated [1,2]

Modifying Circumstances	Probable Organism(s)		Antibiotic Choice(s)	Usual Dosage‡	Cost per Day
ACUTE CYSTITIS FEMALES > 12 YEARS	*E. coli* (80-90%) *S. saprophyticus* Other Gram -ve bacilli	***FIRST LINE***	**TMP/SMX** [2]	2 tabs BID or 1 DS tab BID	$0.08 - $0.24
			Trimethoprim [2]	100 mg BID or 200 mg once daily	$0.51 - $0.53
			Nitrofurantoin [3]	50-100 mg QID or Macrobid 100 mg BID	$0.58 - $0.77 Macrobid: $1.34
			Fosfomycin	Single dose (3 g) dissolved in 1/2 cup of cold water	$24.00
		SECOND LINE	**Amoxicillin** [4]	500 mg TID	$1.73
			Norfloxacin	400 mg BID	$1.09
			Ciprofloxacin [5,6]	250 mg BID or 500 mg (extended release) once daily	$1.24 - $3.08
		THIRD LINE	**Cephalexin**	250-500 mg QID	$0.90 - $1.80
			Levofloxacin [5]	250 mg once daily	$1.20

1) Acute cystitis is characterized by a normal genitourinary tract, limited morbidity, consistent microbiological spectrum. **If further resistance among uropathogens is to be limited, treatment strategies that reduce unnecessary antibiotic use need to be encouraged. The best indicators that an antibiotic is warranted are classic symptoms (dysuria, frequency, urgency) plus pyuria** (Stamm 1993; McIsaac 2007). There is no advantage in routinely sending midstream urine samples for testing (Little 2010). Urine culture is not generally recommended unless failure to respond to empiric therapy or early (< 1 month) recurrence.

2) **Duration of therapy: 3 day therapy for** TMP/SMX, TMP and quinolones. Alternatives to TMP/SMX should be considered when local resistance is anticipated to be > 20%. **5 day therapy for** nitrofurantoin (Gupta 2007). **7 day therapy for** amoxicillin, cephalexin and in women where symptoms last > 7 days or nursing home population.

3) Macro-crystals may be better tolerated than micro-crystalline nitrofurantoin. Nitrofurantoin demonstrated equivalent clinical cures rates compared to TMP/SMX (Gupta 2011). Nitrofurantoin should not be used in infants < 1 month of age or in renal failure (CrCl < 60 mL/min).

4) Amoxicillin is not first choice since 40% of bacteria are resistant; less effective with a cure rate of 60-80% reported; seven days of therapy are required if amoxicillin is used (Gupta 2011; Zhanel 2006).

5) Due to the importance of these fluoroquinolones (FQs) for other indications and concern of developing resistance with overuse, these agents should be reserved for severe situations (Adam 2009; Chen 1999) or if patient is allergic or intolerant to other therapies. Patients who have previously been treated with these FQs may be at a significantly increased risk of contracting community-acquired *E.coli* UTIs that are quinolone (and frequently multi-drug) resistant. However, norfloxacin was not found to select for quinolone-resistant-*E. coli*. Previous quinolone use is also a strong risk factor for infection with a TMP/SMX resistant gram-negative uropathogen. Hence, a recent exposure to FQs and/or a history of recurrent UTI strongly suggest an alternative antibacterial treatment should be used (Hooton 2003, 2004; Karlowsky 2006).

6) Ciprofloxacin has activity vs *Pseudomonas aeruginosa* and should be reserved for this.

References: Adam 2009; Blondeau 2004; Chen 1999; Czaja 2006; Epp 2010; Falagas 2010; Ferry 2004; Fihn 2003; Fitzgerald 2003; Grabe 2011; Gupta 2007, 2011; Hooton 2001, 2003, 2004, 2005, 2012; Karlowsky 2006, 2011; Killgore 2004; Little 2010; McIsaac 2002; Metlay 2003; Moura 2009; Nicolle 2002, 2003, 2006(a), 2008(a, b); O'Donnell 2002; Sanchez 2012; Sheffield 2005; SIGN 2006; Stamm 1993; Vogel 2004; Wagenlehner 2011; Zalmanovici 2010; Zhanel 2006.

Modifying Circumstances	Probable Organism(s)	Antibiotic Choice(s)		Usual Dosage‡	Cost per Day

Recurrent Cystitis – Female [1]

Modifying Circumstances	Probable Organism(s)	Antibiotic Choice(s)		Usual Dosage‡	Cost per Day
EARLY RECURRENCE < 1 MONTH [2]	E. coli S. saprophyticus Other Gram -ve bacilli	FIRST LINE	TMP/SMX [3]	2 tabs BID or 1 DS tab BID	$0.08 - $0.24
			Trimethoprim [3]	100 mg BID or 200 mg once daily	$0.51
			Nitrofurantoin [4]	50-100 mg QID or Macrobid 100 mg BID	$0.58 - $0.77 Macrobid: $1.34
		SECOND LINE	Norfloxacin	400 mg BID	$1.09
			Levofloxacin	250 mg once daily	$1.20
			Ciprofloxacin [5, 6]	250 mg BID or 500 mg (extended release) once daily	$1.24 - $3.08
		THIRD LINE	Cephalexin [7]	250-500 mg QID	$1.80
PROPHYLAXIS OF FREQUENT RECURRENCE (TWO OR MORE EPISODES IN 6 MONTHS OR 3 OR MORE EPISODES IN A YEAR) [8, 9, 10]		FIRST LINE	TMP/SMX [3]	1 tab or ½ DS tab qhs 3 times weekly or post-coital	$0.02 - $0.12
			Trimethoprim [3]	100 mg qhs or post-coital	$0.25
			Nitrofurantoin [4]	50 mg or Macrobid 100 mg qhs or post-coital	$0.14
		SECOND LINE	Cephalexin [7]	125-250 mg qhs or post-coital	$0.11 - $0.23
			Norfloxacin	200 mg every other day or 3 times weekly or post-coital	$0.55
			Fosfomycin	3 g dissolved in 1/2 cup of cold water once every 10 days	$24.00 every 10 days

Continued ...

TMP/SMX = Trimethoprim / Sulfamethoxazole

‡ Common oral dosage ranges are provided unless otherwise stated. Consult the drug monograph for details on age and condition-specific dosing.

Recurrent Cystitis – Female

1) **Culture** re-assess for upper urinary tract infection. Probiotics cannot be recommended as a proven therapy for prevention of urinary tract infections (Epp 2010).

2) Re-treat for 7 to 14 days.

3) Long term low dose TMP/SMX usually does not result in an increase of resistant flora. Alternatives to TMP/SMX should be considered when local resistance is anticipated to be > 20%.

4) Macro-crystals may be better tolerated than micro-crystalline nitrofurantoin. Nitrofurantoin should not be used in infants < 1 month of age.

5) Due to the importance of these fluoroquinolones (FQs) for other indications and concern of developing resistance with overuse, these agents need to be held in reserve for severe situations (Adam 2009; Chen 1999). Patients who have previously been treated with these FQs may be at significantly increased risk of contracting community-acquired *E.coli* UTIs that are quinolone (and frequently multi-drug) resistant. However, norfloxacin was not found to select for quinolone-resistant *E. coli*. In addition, previous quinolone use can be a strong risk factor for infection with a TMP/SMX resistant gram-negative uropathogen. Hence, a recent exposure to FQs and/or a history of recurrent UTI strongly suggest an alternative antibacterial treatment (e.g., nitrofurantoin, cephalosporin, fosfomycin) should be used (Hooton 2003, 2004; Karlowsky 2006; Killgore 2004; Metlay 2003).

6) Ciprofloxacin has activity vs *Pseudomonas aeruginosa*.

7) Cephalexin is not generally recommended, but has a role in treating pregnant women because of safety.

8) An alternative strategy for recurrent infections is short course (e.g., 3 days), self-treatment upon the appearance of symptoms (Hooton 2012)

9) **Drug choice for recurrent infection** should be based on cultures. Consider prophylaxis using continuous low dose or post-coital antibiotics if identified with intercourse. Methenamine mandelate (1 g QID) can also be considered for prophylaxis or suppressive treatment of frequently occurring infections, if available. Patient should be re-assessed following six months of therapy. About 50% of women may experience recurrence by 3 months after discontinuation of the prophylactic antimicrobial. If this occurs, prophylaxis may be reinstituted for as long as 1-2 years and remain effective (Nicolle 2008). Women having frequent recurrences, despite prophylaxis, may require genitourinary investigation. The role of topical estrogens for post-menopausal women in preventing urinary infection remains controversial.

10) Based on an up-dated Cochrane review cranberry juice cannot currently be recommended for the prevention of UTIs. Other preparations (such as cranberry powders) need to be standardised before being evaluated in clinical studies or recommended for use (Jepson 2012).

References: Adam 2009; Chen 1999; Epp 2010; Falagas 2006; Grabe 2011; Gupta 2001; Hooton 2003, 2004; 2012; Jepson 2008, 2012; Karlowsky 2006; Killgore 2004; Kontiokari 2001; Lee 2012; Metlay 2003; Nicolle 2002, 2003, 2008(b); O'Donnell 2002; Regier 2002; Reid 2006; Rudenko 2005; Sanford 2012; Stamm 1993; Stothers 2002.

Modifying Circumstances	Probable Organism(s)	Antibiotic Choice(s)	Usual Dosage‡	Cost per Day

Asymptomatic Bacteriuria [1, 2]

		SCREEN / TREAT ONLY DURING PREGNANCY AND/OR PRE-OP GENITOURINARY PROCEDURES		
E.coli (60-70%) Gram -ve bacilli Group B Strep.	**FIRST LINE**	Amoxicillin	500 mg TID	$1.03
		Nitrofurantoin [3, 4]	50-100 mg QID or Macrobid 100 mg BID	$0.07 - $0.08 Macrobid: $1.24
		TMP/SMX [5]	2 tabs BID or 1 DS tab BID	$0.08 - $0.24
		Trimethoprim [5]	100 mg BID or 200 mg once daily	$0.51 - $0.53
	SECOND LINE	Cephalexin [6]	250-500 mg QID	$1.80
		Amoxicillin/Clavulanate	500 mg TID or 875 mg BID	$1.11 - $2.00
		Norfloxacin [7]	400 mg BID	$1.09
		Levofloxacin [7]	250 mg once daily	$1.20

1) **EXCEPT during pregnancy and/or pre-operative genitourinary (GU) procedures, there are NO indications for screening or therapy for asymptomatic UTI (including in the elderly).**
   GU: Initiate antibiotic therapy immediately before the procedure and continue only for its duration, unless indwelling catheter remains in place.
   Pregnancy: Screen with urine culture at 12-16 weeks' gestation or at the first prenatal visit, if later. If positive, treat with 3-7 day antibiotic course. Perform a follow-up culture and retreat if necessary (Lin 2008; Nicolle 2005(b)).
2) **Overtreatment of asymptomatic urinary infection in the institutionalized elderly and long-term care facility residents is a serious concern.** Positive urine cultures are virtually always associated with pyuria and neither is sufficient for diagnosis or treatment of UTI (Nicolle 2009). See page 71 for treatment of UTI in Nursing Home/LTC patients.
3) Macro-crystals may be better tolerated than micro-crystalline nitrofurantoin. Nitrofurantoin is relatively contraindicated in renal failure (CrCl< 60 mL/min).
4) **Nitrofurantoin is contraindicated in pregnant patients at term (36-42 weeks gestation), during labour and in neonates due to the possibility of hemolytic anemia.**
5) **Avoid trimethoprim and TMP/SMX during the first trimester because of concerns that trimethoprim may limit the availability of folic acid to the fetus and lead to fetal abnormalities. Avoid the use of TMP/SMX during the last six weeks of pregnancy as sulfonamides may displace bilirubin from albumin binding sites causing kernicterus in infants, especially if preterm.** Alternatives to TMP/SMX should be considered when local resistance is anticipated to be > 20%.
6) Cephalexin is not generally recommended, but has a role in treating pregnant women because of safety.
7) It is generally recommended that fluoroquinolones be avoided during pregnancy; especially in the first trimester, as safer alternatives are available; only use if potential benefit justifies risk to the fetus (CPS 2011). For more information consult www.motherisk.org.

References: Colgan 2006; CPS 2011; Dairiki Shortliffe 2002; Epp 2010; Gomolin 2002; Grabe 2011; Gupta 2002; Lin 2008; Macejko 2007; Nicolle 1999, 2002, 2003, 2005(b), 2006(b), 2009; O'Donnell 2002; Shrim 2007; Smaill 2003, 2007; Walker 2000.

Modifying Circumstances	Probable Organism(s)		Antibiotic Choice(s)	Usual Dosage‡	Cost per Day

Acute Cystitis in Pregnant Women [1, 2]

Modifying Circumstances	Probable Organism(s)		Antibiotic Choice(s)	Usual Dosage‡	Cost per Day
	E. coli Klebsiella Proteus Enterococci	**FIRST LINE**	**Cephalexin**	250-500 mg QID	$1.80
			Amoxicillin [3]	500 mg TID	$1.03
			Nitrofurantoin [4]	50-100 mg QID	$0.07 - $0.08
				OR	
				Macrobid 100 mg BID	Macrobid: $1.24
			Fosfomycin	Single dose (3 g) dissolved in 1/2 cup of cold water	$24.00
		SECOND LINE	**TMP/SMX** [5]	2 tabs BID or 1 DS tab BID	$0.08 - $0.24
			Trimethoprim [5]	100 mg BID or 200 mg once daily	$0.51 - $0.53

1) Do monthly follow-up cultures in pregnant women who are susceptible to recurrence. For treatment of pyelonephritis in pregnancy, use ceftriaxone 1-2 g q24h.

2) **Duration of treatment: A three-day** course of therapy for TMP/SMX and trimethoprim is usually sufficient, but follow-up culture should be obtained. Nitrofurantoin should be used for 5 days and amoxicillin and cephalexin for 7 days.

3) Because of high rates of amoxicillin resistance in community *E. coli*, use amoxicillin only after lab confirmation that the implicated bacteria are susceptible (Zhanel 2006). Amoxicillin is highly efficacious for group B strep, sensitive gram-positive organisms (e.g., *S. saprophyticus*) and sensitive E. coli strains (Macejko 2007; Mittal 2005; Grabe 2009; Shrim 2007). When treating with amoxicillin, the duration should be for 7 days.

4) **Nitrofurantoin is contraindicated in pregnant patients at term (36-42 weeks gestation), during labour and in neonates due to the possibility of hemolytic anemia.** Macro-crystals may be better tolerated than micro-crystalline nitrofurantoin.

5) **Avoid trimethoprim and TMP/SMX during the first trimester because of concerns that trimethoprim may limit the availability of folic acid to the fetus and lead to fetal abnormalities. Avoid the use of TMP/SMX during the last six weeks of pregnancy as sulfonamides may displace bilirubin from albumin binding sites causing kernicterus in infants, especially if preterm.** Alternatives to TMP/SMX should be considered when local resistance is anticipated to be > 20%.

References: Briggs 2008; Crider 2009; Delzell 2000; Estebanez 2009; EUR 2009; Grabe 2011; Lee 2008; Macejko 2007; Mittal 2005; MotheRisk 2008; Nicolle 2002, 2003; O'Donnell 2002; Shrim 2007; Smaill 2003; Usta 2011; Vazquez 2011; Zhanel 2006.

TMP/SMX = Trimethoprim / Sulfamethoxazole   © 2013 Anti-infective Review Panel

‡ Common oral dosage ranges are provided unless otherwise stated. Consult the drug monograph for details on age and condition-specific dosing. **Page 69**

Modifying Circumstances	Probable Organism(s)		Antibiotic Choice(s)	Usual Dosage‡	Cost per Day

Acute Urinary Tract Infection – Children [1, 2, 3]

Modifying Circumstances	Probable Organism(s)		Antibiotic Choice(s)	Usual Dosage‡	Cost per Day
	E. coli Enterobacter Proteus Enterococcus	**FIRST LINE**	TMP/SMX [4]	5-10 mg/kg/day trimethoprim divided q12h	$0.02 - $0.03/kg
			Nitrofurantoin [5]	5-7 mg/kg/day divided q6h	$0.03 - $0.04/kg
		SECOND LINE	Amoxicillin [6]	40 mg/kg/day divided q8h	$0.02/kg
			Cephalexin	25-50 mg/kg/day divided q6h	$0.03 - $0.07/kg
			Trimethoprim [7]	4 mg/kg/day divided q12h	
		THIRD LINE	Cefixime	8 mg/kg/day divided q12-24h	$0.19/kg
			Amoxicillin/Clavulanate	40 mg/kg/day amoxicillin divided BID	$0.07/kg

1) UTI is a relatively common infection that can be easily missed in young children; it also may be difficult to differentiate between upper and lower UTI. Classic symptoms are present in older children but often absent in infants, toddlers and preschoolers. Infants have nonspecific symptoms of poor feeding, irritability or fever that may be combined with emesis or abdominal pain. Older infants and toddlers experience vomiting, abdominal pain, urinary retention, back pain, dysuria, frequency, new-onset incontinence or suprapubic tenderness. A previous history of UTI or lack of circumcision are also predisposing factors. Reassess if still unwell after 24-48 hours (Baumer 2007).

2) The use of fluoroquinolones in children remains relatively contraindicated in children < 12 years of age except in life-threatening or extraordinary circumstances (e.g., multidrug resistant bacteria); if fluoroquinolones are considered, consultation with an infectious disease specialist or urologist is suggested, unless the patient is infected with *Pseudomonas aeruginosa*.

3) Patients who are toxic-appearing, dehydrated, or unable to retain oral intake (including medications) should receive antimicrobials parenterally with aminoglycosides and/or ß-lactams (such as ampicillin) until they are able to retain oral fluids and medications. Only a minority of children with a UTI have an underlying urological disorder, but when present such a disorder can cause considerable morbidity. Imaging studies (VCUG, Ultrasound, DMSA scan) are indicated for a child with (1) pyelonephritis; (2) first UTI in a boy of any age; (3) first UTI in a girl < 3 years of age; (4) second UTI in a girl > 3 years of age; (5) first UTI in a child of any age with a family history of UTIs, abnormalities of the urinary tract, an abnormal voiding pattern, hypertension or poor growth (Hoberman 2003; Grabe 2009).

4) Alternatives to TMP/SMX should be considered when local resistance is anticipated to be > 20%.

5) Nitrofurantoin is not active against *P. aeruginosa* or certain strains of *Klebsiella* and *Proteus*. Macro-crystals may be better tolerated than micro-crystalline nitrofurantoin. It should not be used in infants < 1 month of age.

6) Amoxicillin is not recommended for short course therapy due to a high percentage of resistant organisms. Short course therapy is not effective for children under 5 years of age due to a high incidence of reflux.

7) Trimethoprim is not available in liquid form but may be compounded.

References: Bachur 2004; Bauer 2008; Baumer 2007; Chang 2006; Conway 2007; Craig 2009; Dairiki Shortliffe 2002; Fitzgerald 2007; Forsythe 2007; Grabe 2011; Hoberman 2003; Hodson 2003; Koyle 2003; Mori 2007; Murray 2007; NICE 2007; Riccabona 2003; Shah 2005; Shaikh 2007; Tran 2001; Williams 2009; Zorc 2005.

Urinary Tract Infections in Nursing Home/Long Term Care[1, 2, 3]

Modifying Circumstances	Probable Organism(s)		Antibiotic Choice(s)	Usual Dosage‡	Cost per Day
ASYMPTOMATIC BACTERIURIA [1]			NO ANTIBIOTIC INDICATED		
SYMPTOMATIC [2,3]	E. coli Gram -ve bacilli Group B Strep. Enterococcus	FIRST LINE	TMP/SMX	2 tabs BID or 1 DS tab BID	$0.08 - $0.24
			Trimethoprim	100 mg BID or 200 mg once daily	$0.51 - $0.53
			Nitrofurantoin [4, 5]	50-100 mg QID or Macrobid 100 mg BID	$0.58 - $0.77 Macrobid: $1.34
			Amoxicillin [4]	500 mg TID	$1.03
		SECOND LINE	Ciprofloxacin	250 mg BID or 500 mg (extended release) once daily	$1.24 - $3.08
			Levofloxacin	250 mg once daily	$1.20
			Amoxicillin/Clavulanate	500 mg TID or 875 mg BID	$1.11 - $2.00

1) Urinary tract infection (UTI) is the most common infection in long-term care residents. One third of prescriptions for presumed UTI in this population are for asymptomatic bacteriuria or the presence of bacteria in the urine in the absence of urinary symptoms (Loeb 2005). **Routine screening and treatment for asymptomatic bacteriuria in nursing home residents is not recommended** (Loeb 2002; Juthani-Metha 2007). While there is a very high prevalence of asymptomatic urinary infection (15-30% of men and 25-50% of women have positive urine cultures), treating these patients, whether or not accompanied by pyuria, is not beneficial and may be harmful. (Nicolle 1997, 2009). Diligent hygiene is very important in preventing infection in incontinent patients.

2) **Minimum criteria for initiating antibiotics for an indication of UTI in residents with no indwelling urinary catheter or residents maintained with intermittent catheterization or condom catheter:** Acute dysuria alone OR fever AND at least one of the following: new or worsening urgency, frequency, suprapubic pain, gross hematuria, costovertebral angle tenderness or urinary incontinence. **Minimum criteria for a suspected UTI in patients with an indwelling catheter:** Presence of at least one of the following: fever, new costovertebral tenderness, rigors with or without identified cause or new onset of delirium (Loeb 2001). Change in character of the urine or in mental status are not, in the absence of concomitant localizing genitourinary symptoms (lower tract irritation, increased frequency of incontinence and fever) a reliable predictor. Acute symptoms may be difficult to recognize because of impaired communication, dementia or comorbid illnesses. Non-specific presentations (fever or chills, malaise, dehydration, syncope or changes in behaviour, gait or falls, voiding pattern, functional status) should not be interpreted as symptomatic urinary infection in residents without a chronic indwelling catheter (Bentley 2000; Loeb 2001; Nicolle 2009; Orr 1996). **A urine specimen for culture should always be obtained before initiating antimicrobial therapy.** Given the high prevalence of bacteriuria, a positive urine culture is not diagnostic for symptomatic urinary infection.

3) Generally 7 day treatment is required. For women presenting with lower tract symptoms, 3 days of ciprofloxacin 250 mg BID is as effective as 7 days of therapy and is associated with fewer adverse effects (Vogel 2004). For individuals presenting with fever or more severe systemic symptoms, 10-14 days of therapy is recommended. The only current indication for prophylactic antimicrobial therapy is for bacteriuric subjects before they undergo an invasive urologic procedure.

4) Amoxicillin may be used for susceptible organisms but resistance is approximately 40% (Zhanel 2006). Resistance rate to nitrofurantoin in Canada is 21% in nursing home population, although it is low (6-8%) in other clinical settings (Laupland 2007). Cephalexin can also be used for susceptible strains.

5) Nitrofurantoin is relatively contraindicated in renal impairment (CrCl< 60mL/min).

References: Beier 1999; Bentley 2000; Juthani-Metha 2007 (a,b); Laupland 2007; Loeb 2001, 2002, 2005; Lutters 2007; Monette 2007; Nicole 1997, 2009; Orr 1996; TOP 2010; Vogel 2004; Zhanel 2006.

TMP/SMX = Trimethoprim / Sulfamethoxazole

‡ Common oral dosage ranges are provided unless otherwise stated. Consult the drug monograph for details on age and condition-specific dosing.

Modifying Circumstances	Probable Organism(s)		Antibiotic Choice(s)	Usual Dosage‡	Cost per Day

Complicated Urinary Tract Infection – Adult[1, 2]

Modifying Circumstances	Probable Organism(s)		Antibiotic Choice(s)	Usual Dosage‡	Cost per Day
ORAL THERAPY MILD TO MODERATE	E. coli (50%) P. mirabilis (20%) Enterococci Klebsiella Proteus P. aeruginosa Other Gram -ve bacilli	FIRST LINE	TMP/SMX [3]	2 tabs BID or 1 DS tab BID	$0.08 - $0.24
			Trimethoprim [3]	200 mg BID	$0.53
			Nitrofurantoin [4]	50 - 100 mg QID or Macrobid 100 mg BID	$0.07 - $0.08 Macrobid: $1.24
			Norfloxacin	400 mg BID	$1.09
			Ciprofloxacin [5, 6]	500 mg BID or 1 g (extended release) once daily	$1.40 - $3.08
			Levofloxacin [6]	500 mg once daily x 10 days or 750 mg x 5 days	$1.37 - 6.54
		SECOND LINE [7]	Amoxicillin/Clavulanate	500 mg TID or 875 mg BID	$1.11 - $2.00
PARENTERAL THERAPY [8] SEVERE		FIRST LINE	Ampicillin IV	1 g q6h	
			PLUS ANY ONE of the following:		
			Amikacin IV [9]	15 - 20 mg/kg q24h	IV costs vary according to jurisdiction and/or contract pricing.
			Gentamicin IV [9]	4 - 7 mg/kg q24h	
			Tobramycin IV [9]	4 - 7 mg/kg q24h	
		SECOND LINE	Cefotaxime IV	1 - 2 g q12h	
			Ceftriaxone IV/IM	1 - 2 g q24h	
			Ciprofloxacin IV [5, 6]	200 - 400 mg q12h	
			Levofloxacin IV [6]	250 mg q24h	
			Ticarcillin/Clavulanate	3.1 g q4-6h	
			Piperacillin / Tazobactam	3 g / 0.375 g q6h	
		THIRD LINE	Ceftazidime IV [10]	1 - 2 g q8h	
			Imipenem / Cilastatin IV	500 mg q6h	
			Meropenem	500 - 1000 mg q8h	

Continued ...

TMP/SMX = Trimethoprim / Sulfamethoxazole

‡ Common oral dosage ranges are provided unless otherwise stated. Consult the drug monograph for details on age and condition-specific dosing.

Complicated Urinary Tract Infection – Adult

1) **Culture required before antibiotic therapy. Duration of treatment:** if lower tract (bladder) mild to moderate symptoms, treat for 7-10 days; if upper tract (kidney) symptoms or systemic (e.g., high fever, sepsis, vomiting), treat 10-14 days. Short course therapy (e.g., 3 days) is not recommended (Nicolle 2005(a)).

2) Complicated UTI includes patients with structural or functional abnormalities such as: obstruction, chronic catheter, spinal cord injury, etc. or any UTI in men. It is characterized by mixed bacteriology and, generally, more resistant organisms. Investigate any underlying causes; with persistent abnormalities recurrent infection is common (50% by 6 weeks post-therapy). Patients with catheters should not be treated unless there is evidence of systemic disease.

3) Alternatives to TMP/SMX should be considered when local resistance is anticipated to be > 20%.

4) Nitrofurantoin is not active against *P. aeruginosa* or certain strains of *Klebsiella* and *Proteus* species. While it can be used in certain circumstances (e.g., prophylaxis of complicated UTI) it is not well absorbed in tissue and should not be used in upper tract infection. It is rarely effective if UTI is associated with obstruction, foreign body or tissue infection. Macro-crystals may be better tolerated than micro-crystalline nitrofurantoin. Nitrofurantoin is relatively contraindicated in patients with renal failure (CrCl < 60 ml/min).

5) Ciprofloxacin has activity vs *Pseudomonas aeruginosa*.

6) Due to the importance of these fluoroquinolones (FQs) for other indications and concern of developing resistance with overuse, these agents need to be held in reserve for severe situations (Adam 2009; Chen 1999).

7) Cephalexin 500 mg QID and cefixime 400 mg once daily are also reasonable alternative therapies.

8) IV therapy is indicated for the patients who are unable to tolerate oral therapy, have impaired GI absorption, have hemodynamic instability, or if the infecting organism is resistant to oral agents. If initiating parenteral treatment, switch to oral therapy after 72-96 hours or when clinically appropriate and when culture and sensitivity results are available to direct choice.

9) For more information on aminoglycoside dosing, see page 109.

10) Ceftazidime should only be used if *P. aeruginosa* is a consideration.

References: Grabe 2009, 2011; Klimberg 1998; Neal 2008; Nicolle 2002, 2003, 2005(a); O'Donnell 2002; Petersen 2008; Regier 2002; Rubenstein 2003; Schaeffer 2002; SIGN 2006; Wagenlehner 2006(a), 2009.

Modifying Circumstances	Probable Organism(s)		Antibiotic Choice(s)	Usual Dosage‡	Cost per Day

Pyelonephritis [1]

Modifying Circumstances	Probable Organism(s)		Antibiotic Choice(s)	Usual Dosage‡	Cost per Day
UNCOMPLICATED NON-OBSTRUCTION MILD [2]	E. coli (90%) K. pneumoniae P. mirabilis	FIRST LINE	TMP/SMX [3]	2 tabs BID or 1 DS tab BID	$0.08 - $0.24
			Trimethoprim [3]	100 mg BID or 200 mg once daily	$0.51 - $0.53
			Norfloxacin	400 mg BID	$1.09
			Ciprofloxacin [4]	500 mg BID or 1 g (extended release) once daily	$1.40 - $3.08
			Levofloxacin	500 mg once daily x 10 days or 750 mg once daily x 5 days	$1.37 - $6.55
		SECOND LINE	Amoxicillin/Clavulanate	500 mg TID or 875 mg BID	$1.11 - $2.00
SEVERE [5]		FIRST LINE	Gentamicin IV [6] ±	4 - 7 mg/kg q24h	
			Ampicillin IV [7]	1 - 2 g q4-6h	
		SECOND LINE	Ciprofloxacin IV	400 mg q12h	IV costs vary according to jurisdiction and/or contract pricing.
			Levofloxacin IV	250 - 500 mg q24h	
			[Cefotaxime IV OR	1 - 2 g q12h	
			Ceftriaxone IV/IM] ±	1 - 2 g q24h	
			Gentamicin IV [6]	4 - 7 mg/kg q24h	
COMPLICATED			See Complicated UTI		

1) **Pre-treatment culture required. Duration of therapy:** Treat with 10-14 day course of therapy unless otherwise indicated. Repeat cultures during follow-up are not recommended for patients who remain asymptomatic (Nicolle 2008). If no clinical improvement is noted or if status worsens after 72 hours of treatment, investigation for complications of renal infection or urinary obstruction should be undertaken (Grabe 2009; Sheffield 2005; Nicolle 2008). For patients who have overt sepsis or those who are unable to tolerate oral medications, hospitalization and IV antibiotics are recommended. Many other oral and IV agents may be effective.

2) Low-grade fever, normal or slightly elevated peripheral leukocyte count without nausea or vomiting.

3) Alternatives to TMP/SMX should be considered when local resistance is anticipated to be > 20%.

4) Ciprofloxacin has activity vs *Pseudomonas aeruginosa*. Ciprofloxacin x 7 days is adequate therapy for less severe presentations.

5) If initiating treatment with parenteral therapy, switch to oral therapy after three or four days if clinically appropriate and when culture and sensitivity results are available to direct therapeutic choice.

6) Tobramycin or amikacin can also be used. For more information on aminoglycoside dosing, see page 109.

7) Diabetics and pregnant women are more susceptible to *Group B Strep.* and require ampicillin to be added.

References: Grabe 2011; Gupta 2011; Hooton 2003, 2012; Nicolle 2008(b,c); Ramakrishnan 2005; Sheffield 2005; Talan2000; Warren 1999.

Modifying Circumstances	Probable Organism(s)	Antibiotic Choice(s)	Usual Dosage‡	Cost per Day

Prostatitis – Acute [1, 2]

Modifying Circumstances	Probable Organism(s)	Antibiotic Choice(s)	Usual Dosage‡	Cost per Day
MOST LIKELY BACTERIAL **MILD TO MODERATE**	E. coli **FIRST** Other **LINE** Gram -ve bacilli S. aureus E. faecalis	**TMP/SMX** [3]	2 tabs BID or 1 DS tab BID	$0.08 - $0.24
		Trimethoprim [3]	200 mg BID	$1.06
		Norfloxacin	400 mg BID	$1.09
		Ofloxacin	300 - 400 mg BID	$3.06
		Levofloxacin	500 mg once daily	$1.37
		Ciprofloxacin [4]	500 mg BID or 1 g (extended release) once daily	$1.40 - $3.08
SEVERE [5]	**FIRST LINE**	**Ampicillin IV**	1 - 2 g q4-6h	$7.60
		OR		
		Ceftriaxone IV	1 - 2 g q12 - 24h	$12.50 - $48.28
		PLUS ANY ONE of the following:		
		Gentamicin IV [6]	4 - 7 mg/kg q24h	80 mg: $3.96
		Tobramycin IV [6]	4 - 7 mg/kg q24h	80 mg: $4.50
		Amikacin IV [6]	15 - 20 mg/kg q24h	250 mg: $31.22

1) Symptoms include acute onset chills, fever, perineal and low back pain, irritative and obstructive voiding. Prostate is tender, swollen, indurated and warm. Voided urine specimen before empiric therapy. If no evidence of improvement after two weeks, then reassess. In older men with relapsing UTI, the prostate is often the source. Prostate massage should be avoided because it is painful and may cause bacteremia (CAN STI 2008). Acute prostatitis, although very rare, can occur in prepubertal boys.

2) Patient may not be able to void, in which case hospitalization and catheterization may be necessary.

3) The current consensus of prostatitis experts is that TMP/SMX and TMP are only indicated once culture results confirm sensitivity (Nickel 2009). Alternatives to TMP/SMX should be considered when local resistance is anticipated to be > 20%.

4) Ciprofloxacin has activity vs *Pseudomonas aeruginosa*.

5) Once acute symptoms have resolved, an additional two to four weeks of oral therapy (based on culture and sensitivity data) is indicated. For patients who cannot tolerate or are allergic to penicillin and/or aminoglycoside, use intravenous ciprofloxacin or levofloxacin.

6) For more information on aminoglycoside dosing, see page 109.

References: BASHH 2008; Benway 2008; CAN STI 2008; Drusano 2000; Grabe 2011; Johns Hopkins 2011; Joly-Guillou 1999; Naber 2001; Nickel 1999, 2000, 2004, 2009; Sobel 2002; Wagenlehner 2006(a), 2007.

Modifying Circumstances	Probable Organism(s)		Antibiotic Choice(s)	Usual Dosage‡	Cost per Day

Prostatitis - Chronic [1, 2]

Modifying Circumstances	Probable Organism(s)		Antibiotic Choice(s)	Usual Dosage‡	Cost per Day
	E. coli Other gram -ve bacilli E. faecalis P. aeruginosa	FIRST LINE	Norfloxacin	400 mg BID	$1.09
			Ofloxacin	300-400 mg BID	$3.06
			Levofloxacin	500 mg once daily	$1.37
			Ciprofloxacin [3]	500 mg BID or 1 g (extended release) once daily	$1.40 - $3.08
		SECOND LINE	TMP/SMX [4]	2 tabs BID or 1DS tab BID	$0.08 - $0.24
			Trimethoprim [4]	200 mg BID	$1.06

1) This is an uncommon and very difficult diagnostic category; prevalence increases with age. Symptoms vary but include dysuria, other voiding complaints, ejaculatory or genital pain; some patients may be asymptomatic and prostate examination is usually normal (CAN STI 2008). Chronic bacterial prostatitis is characterized by recurrent episodes of bacteriuria due to the same organism; chronic non-bacterial prostatitis is of unknown etiology and does not respond to antibiotics. Generally, antibiotics do not have a role unless abscess or positive urine culture is present. When treating chronic prostatitis, cultures may be negative but clinical presentation significant; best to treat with syndrome approach. If there is no response in four to six weeks, chronic patients should be referred to a urologist (Benway 2008). Chronic cases are less likely to be true bacterial prostatitis.

2) Alpha-blockers and antibiotics, as well as combinations of these therapies, appear to achieve the greatest improvement in clinical symptom scores compared with placebo (Anothaisintawee 2011). Fluoroquinolones have been shown to have comparable bacterial eradication and clinical cure rates that are superior to TMP/SMX and trimethoprim (Naber 1999; Nickel 2004; Schaeffer 2006).

3) Ciprofloxacin has activity vs *Pseudomonas aeruginosa*.

4) Alternatives to TMP/SMX should be considered when local resistance is anticipated to be > 20%.

References: Anothaisintawee 2011; BASHH 2008; Benway 2008; Bjerklund 1998; Bundrick 2003; CAN STI 2008; Drusano 2000; Grabe 2011; Habermacher 2006; Joly-Guillou 1999; Naber 1999, 2001; Nickel 1999, 2000, 2003, 2004, 2005; Schaeffer 2006; Sobel 2002.

Modifying Circumstances	Probable Organism(s)		Antibiotic Choice(s)	Usual Dosage‡	Cost per Day

Epididymitis [1, 2, 3, 4]

Modifying Circumstances	Probable Organism(s)		Antibiotic Choice(s)	Usual Dosage‡	Cost per Day
> 35 YEARS	E. coli Other Gram -ve bacilli	FIRST LINE	Ofloxacin [5]	300 mg BID	10 days: $30.60
			Ciprofloxacin [5]	500 mg BID or 1 g (extended release) once daily	10 days: $14.00 - $30.80
			Levofloxacin [5]	500 mg once daily	10 days: $13.70
≤ 35 YEARS OR Multiple sex partners	N. gonorrhoeae C. trachomatis	FIRST LINE	[Cefixime	800 mg orally in a single dose	$7.08
			OR		
			Ceftriaxone IM]	250-500 mg single dose	$3.95
			PLUS		
			Doxycycline	100 mg BID	10 days: $11.70
		SECOND LINE	Ciprofloxacin [5]	500 mg single dose **Not approved for children**	$0.70
			Levofloxacin [5]	500 mg single dose **Not approved for children < 18 years**	$1.37
			Ceftriaxone IM	250-500 mg single dose	$3.95
			ANY ONE of the above PLUS ONE of the following:		
			Azithromycin	1 g single dose	$5.23
			Doxycycline	100 mg BID	10 days: $11.70

1) Epididymitis in sexually active men < 35 years is most often caused by *C. trachomatis* or *N. gonorrhoeae*. The non-sexually transmitted epididymitis (associated with UTIs) occurs more often in men > 35 years, those who have undergone urinary tract surgery or instrumentation, and/or those who have urinary tract abnormalities. In patients > 35 years of age, while *E. coli* is the predominant pathogen, *C. trachomatis* or *N. gonorrhoeae* should still be considered. **Epididymitis can be secondary to prostatitis and may require up to 6 weeks of therapy.**

2) Presents as an inflammation of the epididymis manifested by acute onset of unilateral testicular pain and swelling, often with tenderness of the epididymis and vas deferens and occasionally with erythema and edema of the overlying skin. When epididymitis is accompanied by urethral discharge, it is presumed to be a sexually acquired infection. The urethritis, however may be asymptomatic and therefore overlooked. If no polymorphonuclear cells are detected or there is a failure to improve within 3 days of initiation of antimicrobial therapy, reevaluate. It is important to consider non-infectious causes of scrotal swelling (i.e., trauma, torsion of the testicle and tumour). The differential diagnosis includes tumor, abscess, infarction, testicular cancer, TB and fungal epididymitis. Torsion of the testicle is a surgical emergency which should be suspected when onset of scrotal pain is sudden.

3) All sexual partners of patients with sexually acquired epididymitis should be evaluated (CAN STI 2008).

4) **Duration of therapy:** 10-14 days unless otherwise indicated. An anti-inflammatory may be indicated.

5) Ciprofloxacin can be considered if *Pseudomonas* is documented or suspected. Due to increased resistance, quinolones should be avoided for empiric therapy of gonococcal infections and should only be considered as an alternative treatment option if susceptibility is demonstrated. In 2006 in Ontario, about one-third (28%) of *N. gonorrhoeae* isolates were resistant to quinolones (Ota 2009). Quinolones should not be used if there is a possibility the infection was acquired in places known to have increased resistance (e.g., South East Asia). If they are used in such cases, a test-of-cure is recommended.

References: BASHH 2010; CAN STI 2008; CDC 2010; Horner 2001; Kropp 2007; Ota 2009; Smith 2007; Tapsall 2009; Workowski 2008.

‡ Common oral dosage ranges are provided unless otherwise stated. Consult the drug monograph for details on age and condition-specific dosing.

Modifying Circumstances	Probable Organism(s)		Antibiotic Choice(s)	Usual Dosage‡	Cost per Day

Pelvic Inflammatory Disease (PID) – Outpatient [1, 2, 3]

Modifying Circumstances	Probable Organism(s)		Antibiotic Choice(s)	Usual Dosage‡	Cost per Day
MILD TO MODERATE PRESENTATION	N. gonorrhoeae C. trachomatis E. coli Anaerobes S. agalactiae H. influenzae	FIRST LINE	Cefixime [4]	800 mg single dose	$7.08
			OR		
			Ceftriaxone IM [4]	250-500 mg single dose	$3.95
			ONE of the above PLUS:		
			Doxycycline [3]	100 mg BID for 14 days	14 days: $16.38
			±		
			Metronidazole [5]	500 mg BID for 14 days	14 days: $11.90
		SECOND LINE	Ofloxacin [4, 6]	400 mg BID for 14 days	14 days: $42.84
			OR		
			Levofloxacin [4, 6]	500 mg once daily for 14 days	14 days: $19.18
			ONE of the above ±		
			Metronidazole [5]	500 mg BID for 14 days	14 days: $11.90

1) Reportable to the Medical Officer of Health.
2) All male sex partners should be treated empirically with regimens effective against both C. trachomatis and N.gonorrhoeae if they had sexual contacts with the patient during the 60 days preceding the onset of symptoms, regardless of clinical findings and without waiting for test results (CDC 2010; CAN STI 2010).
3) **Early treatment is essential. All patients treated as outpatients should be re-evaluated 48-72 hours after the initial assessment and if their condition has not improved, they should be admitted to hospital and a specialist consulted.** Women who have had an episode of PID, have a ten-fold increased risk of subsequent PID, an eight-fold increased risk of ectopic pregnancy and a ten-fold increased risk of tubal infertility.

   Symptoms include: lower abdominal pain of recent onset, heavy menstrual, inter-menstrual or post-coital vaginal bleeding, deep dyspareunia, vaginal discharge that is not explained.

   Signs: cervical motion tenderness, adnexal tenderness on bimanual examination (with or without a mass), cervicitis (purulent cervical exudate present in 30% of cases), fever (present in > 40% of PID cases).

   Pregnancy: PID is rare in pregnancy, especially after the 1st trimester. These patients may require hospitalization to consider other diagnoses. The use of tetracyclines is contraindicated in pregnancy. Fluoroquinolones and tetracyclines are contraindicated in lactating women (MotheRisk 2008).

   Patients with IUD: IUD should not be removed until after therapy is initiated and at least 2 doses of antibiotics have been given. If risk of pregnancy is high, consider leaving IUD in place.
4) For patients with contraindications to treatment with cephalosporins or quinolones evidence suggests a short course of azithromycin (250mg daily x 7 days OR 1 g weekly x 14 days) plus metronidazole is effective in producing clinical cure.
5) Add metronidazole for women with adnexal mass formation, tubo-ovarian abscess, peritonitis or increased risk of anaerobes. Metronidazole can be added where there is concern over lack of anaerobic coverage. Metronidazole will effectively treat bacterial vaginosis that is commonly associated with PID (CDC 2006).
6) Quinolones can still be useful in acute PID that does not involve quinolone resistant N. gonorrheae.

References: BASHH 2011; CAN STI 2010; CDC 2010; Haggerty 2007; Ross 2001, 2003, 2006, 2007; Savaris 2007; Smith 2007.

‡ Common oral dosage ranges are provided unless otherwise stated. Consult the drug monograph for details on age and condition-specific dosing.

Vulvovaginitis

NOTES:

- Definition: Inflammation of the vulva, vagina, or both and/or abnormal vaginal discharge not due to cervicitis.
- When there is infectious etiology, vulvovaginitis is caused by a disruption of the normal lactobacilli dominant flora of the vagina.
- Infectious causes of vaginitis/vaginosis include: bacterial vaginosis, candidiasis, *Trichomonas vaginalis* or mixed infections or physiological discharge.
- Non-infectious causes: Excessive physiologic secretions, hypersensitivity (e.g., latex condoms, vaginal douches, soap), multiple dermatologic conditions (e.g., eczema, psoriasis, atrophy), foreign body, trauma, lack of proper vaginal lubrication during intercourse.

Clinical Clues

Etiology	Predisposing Factors	Symptoms	Signs/quality of discharge
Bacterial Vaginosis	• Often absent • More common if sexually active • New sexual partner • IUD use	• Vaginal discharge • Fishy odour • May increase after intercourse • 50% asymptomatic	• Grey to white thin vaginal discharge, often copious • Inflammation and erythema of vagina are unusual in uncomplicated BV
Candidiasis	• Often absent • Current or recent use of antibiotics • Pregnancy • Corticosteroids • Poorly controlled diabetes mellitus • Immunocompromised • More common if sexually active	• Itch • External dysuria • Vaginal discharge • Post-coital dyspareunia • Up to 20% asymptomatic	• White, clumpy adherent vaginal discharge • Erythema and edema of vulva, vagina and/or introitus • Fissures of vulvar epithelium
Trichomoniasis	• Multiple sexual partners	• Profuse vaginal discharge • Itch • Post-coital dyspareunia • Dysuria • 10-50% asymptomatic	• Frothy, off-white/yellow vaginal discharge • Often erythema of vagina and exocervix

References: BASHH 2010; CAN STI 2010; CDC 2010; Majeroni 2007; Prodigy 2007; Smith 2007; Van Vranken 2007.

Modifying Circumstances	Probable Organism(s)	Antibiotic Choice(s)	Usual Dosage‡	Cost per Day

Vaginitis: (Trichomoniasis) [1, 2, 3, 4]

Modifying Circumstances	Probable Organism(s)	Antibiotic Choice(s)	Usual Dosage‡	Cost per Day
TREAT ALL CASES AND THEIR SEXUAL PARTNERS REGARDLESS OF SYMPTOMS	*T. vaginalis*	**FIRST LINE** Metronidazole OR Metronidazole	2 g orally single dose 500 mg BID for 7 days	Treatment: $0.48 7 days: $5.95

1) It is important to rule out cervicitis when diagnosing vaginitis. *T. vaginalis* and HSV are most often sexually transmitted. Up to 50% of patients are asymptomatic.

2) Some guidelines suggest clinicians may defer or not treat asymptomatic pregnant women (CAN STI 2008; CDC 2010).

3) **Pregnancy: Symptomatic** - treat with 2g metronidazole in a single dose; this treatment can be used at any stage of pregnancy. An alternative treatment is metronidazole 500 mg PO bid for 7 days.
   Asymptomatic - treatment not recommended.
   Lactation - metronidazole is not contraindicated during breastfeeding, however, it does enter breast milk and may affect its taste. In lactating women who are administered metronidazole, withholding breastfeeding during treatment and for 12–24 hours after the last dose will reduce the exposure of the infant to metronidazole. Avoid high doses if breastfeeding (BASHH 2007; CAN STI 2010; CDC 2010; Einarson 2000).

4) Intravaginal metronidazole gel is not effective.

References: BASHH 2007; CAN STI 2008; CDC 2010; Cudmore 2004; Einarson 2000; Forna 2007; Gülmezoglu 2003, 2007; Klebanoff 2001; Schwebke 2004; Van Vranken 2007.

Modifying Circumstances	Probable Organism(s)		Antibiotic Choice(s)	Usual Dosage‡	Cost per Day

Bacterial Vaginosis [1, 2, 3]

Modifying Circumstances	Probable Organism(s)		Antibiotic Choice(s)	Usual Dosage‡	Cost per Day
ASYMPTOMATIC	Mixed anaerobic/ aerobic	*FIRST LINE*	Treatment is unnecessary unless high-risk pregnancy (e.g., prior pre-term delivery), prior to IUD insertion, gynecologic surgery, induced abortion, or upper tract instrumentation.		
SYMPTOMATIC No treatment needed for male sexual partner	Overgrowth of *G. vaginalis M. hominis* Anaerobes	*FIRST LINE*	Metronidazole	500 mg BID orally for 7 days	7 days: $5.95
			Metronidazole 0.75% gel	One applicatorful (5 g) intravaginally once nightly for 5 days	45 g: $28.50
			Clindamycin 2% cream	One applicatorful (5 g) intravaginally once nightly for 7 days	40 g: $27.60
		SECOND LINE	Metronidazole [4]	2 g single dose	$0.48
			Clindamycin	300 mg BID for 7 days	7 days: $6.21

1) The characteristic feature of bacterial vaginosis (BV) is that it is a noninflammatory condition of the vaginal flora. BV is linked with gynecological risks which include PID, cervicitis, post-operation infection and other STIs. It is important to rule out cervicitis when diagnosing bacterial vaginosis.
   Asymptomatic BV: Treatment is unnecessary except in cases of high-risk pregnancy (history of preterm delivery), prior to IUD insertion or prior to gynecologic surgery, therapeutic abortion or upper tract instrumentation.
   Recurrent BV: Treat with metronidazole 500 mg orally BID for 10-14 days or metronidazole gel 0.75%, one applicator (5 g) once a day intravaginally for 10 days, followed by suppressive therapy of metronidazole gel twice a week for 4-6 months (CAN STI 2008).

2) **Pregnancy:** BV in pregnancy has been associated with adverse outcomes, therefore all pregnant women with symptomatic BV require treatment (CAN STI 2008). Evidence supports screening and treatment at 12-16 weeks in high-risk pregnancies. In low-risk and asymptomatic pregnant women, screening and treatment has not shown any benefit. Metronidazole use during pregnancy does not appear to increase the rate of major birth defects above the baseline rate of 1% to 3% (Einarson 2000); however, some experts would avoid using oral metronidazole in the first trimester. In the first and second trimester of pregnancy, topical metronidazole can be used instead of oral metronidazole; the applicator should not be used after the 7th month of pregnancy. Oral therapy is recommended during the third trimester of pregnancy to prevent subclinical infection of the chorioamnion. Testing should be repeated after 1 month to ensure that therapy was effective. **Lactation:** Some experts suggest interrupting breastfeeding until 24 hours after completing therapy, since oral metronidazole is excreted into breast milk in relatively large amounts (up to 20%), however there have been no reports of adverse effects on breastfed infants of mothers who took metronidazole (CAN STI 2008; Einarson 2000). Others prefer topical treatment (CAN STI 2008; CDC 2010; Nygren 2008).

3) Lactobacilli preparations (e.g., lactobacillus acidophilus or rhamnosus) are commonly used in the treatment of BV and VVC. There is limited evidence to support the efficacy of these products (CAN STI 2008; Falagas 2007; Ozkinay 2005; Parent 1996; Pirotta 2004; Reid 2003). It cannot yet be concluded definitively that probiotics are useful for this purpose.

4) A single dose of metronidazole has a cure rate of 85% but a higher relapse rate at 1 month (35–50% vs 20–33%) (CAN STI 2008).

References: BASHH 2006; CAN STI 2008; CDC 2010; Einarson 2000, 2002; Falagas 2007; Ferris 1995; Guise 2001; Hanson 2000; Joesoef 1995; Kane 2001; Klebanoff 2003; Livengood 1999; McDonald 2007; McGregor 1994; Nygren 2008; Okun 2005; Ozkinay 2005; Parent 1996; Reid 2003; Senok 2007; Vermeulen 1999.

© 2013 Anti-infective Review Panel

‡ Common oral dosage ranges are provided unless otherwise stated. Consult the drug monograph for details on age and condition-specific dosing. **Page 81**

Modifying Circumstances	Probable Organism(s)	Antibiotic Choice(s)	Usual Dosage‡	Cost per Day

Vulvovaginal Candidiasis (VVC) [1, 2, 3, 4, 5]

Modifying Circumstances	Probable Organism(s)	Antibiotic Choice(s)	Usual Dosage‡	Cost per Day
ASYMPTOMATIC	Candida sp. and other	**FIRST LINE** Treatment is unnecessary		
SYMPTOMATIC		**FIRST LINE** Butoconazole 2% cream	One applicatorful (5 g) Intravaginally single dose	5 g: $17.25
		Clotrimazole	500 mg tab intravaginally single dose OR 200 mg tab intravaginally daily for 3 days	Treatment: $9.06
		Clotrimazole 10% cream	One applicatorful intravaginally single dose	30 g: $5.25
		Clotrimazole 1% cream	One applicatorful intravaginally daily for 6 days	30 g: $6.64
		Clotrimazole 2% cream	One applicatorful intravaginally daily for 3 days	30 g: $13.27
		Miconazole	100 mg ovule suppository intravaginally daily for 7 days OR 400 mg ovule intravaginally daily for 3 days OR 1200 mg ovule intravaginally single dose	Treatment: $9.78 $3.26 $16.49
		Miconazole 2% cream	One applicatorful intravaginally daily for 7 days	35 g: 9.78
		Miconazole 4% cream	One applicatorful Intravaginally daily for 3 days	$18.00
		Fluconazole [4]	150 mg cap single dose (ORAL)	Treatment: $7.29
		Terconazole	80 mg ovule intravaginally daily for 3 days plus 0.8% cream (Dual Pak)	Treatment: $22.15
		Terconazole 0.4% cream	One applicatorful intravaginally daily for 7 days	45 g: $12.27

Continued ...

Vulvovaginal Candidiasis (VVC)

1) It is important to rule out cervicitis when diagnosing vulvovaginal candidiasis. Topical and oral azoles are equally effective with an estimated efficacy of 80-90% (CAN STI 2008; Nurbhai 2007). In most cases, expect resolution of symptoms in 2-3 days. Male sexual partner should only be treated if *Candida balanitis* is present (which is characterized by erythematous areas on the glans in conjunction with pruritus or irritation); use fluconazole 150 mg single dose or miconazole or clotrimazole cream applied BID for 7 days (CAN STI 2008; CDC 2010; Sobel 2004).
   Asymptomatic: Treatment is unnecessary.

2) For intravaginal products, bedtime administration is preferable. Several of these preparations are available as over-the-counter products.

3) Recurrent VVC (4 or more episodes annually) requires investigation for underlying causes (including a vaginal culture) and different therapeutic strategies. Consultation with a colleague experienced in this area may need to be sought. Without maintenance therapy, VVC recurs in 50% of patients within 3 months. Treatment requires induction, usually followed by a 6-month maintenance regimen:
   Induction Treatment: Fluconazole 150 mg orally once every 72 hours for three doses or topical azole for 10-14 days.
   Maintenance therapy: Fluconazole 150 mg orally once a week for 3-6 months. Alternatives: ketoconazole 100 mg orally once a day or itraconazole 200-400 mg orally once a month or clotrimazole 500 mg intravaginally once a month or other topical treatments used intermittently (however, there is limited data for topical regiments).

4) Topical anti-fungal agents are the treatment of choice during pregnancy. Longer treatment for 7 days may be more effective as compared to shorter courses. Oral azoles (e.g., fluconazole) are not recommended during pregnancy (CAN STI 2008; FDA MedWatch 2011).

5) Lactobacilli preparations (e.g., lactobacillus acidophilus or rhamnosus) are commonly used in the treatment of BV and VVC. There is limited evidence to support the efficacy of these products (CAN STI 2008; Falagas 2007; Health Canada 2006; Ozkinay 2005; Parent 1996; Pirotta 2004; Reid 2003). It cannot yet be concluded definitively that probiotics are useful for this purpose.

References: Aleck 1997; BASHH 2007; CAN STI 2008; CDC 2010; Falagas 2007; FDA MedWatch 2011; Health Canada 2006; Jick 1999; Mastroiacovo 1996; Nurbhai 2007; Ozkinay 2005; Parent 1996; Pirotta 2004; Pursley 1996; Reid 2003; Rogers 1998; Sherrard 2001; Sobel 2007; Sorensen 1999; Watson 2003; Young 2003.

Modifying Circumstances	Probable Organism(s)	Antibiotic Choice(s)	Usual Dosage‡	Cost per Day

Urethritis – Gonococcal [1, 2, 3]

Modifying Circumstances	Probable Organism(s)	Antibiotic Choice(s)	Usual Dosage‡	Cost per Day
ADOLESCENTS AND ADULTS ≥ 9 YEARS	N. gonorrhoeae C. trachomatis[2] **FIRST LINE**	**Cefixime**	400-800 mg single dose	$3.48 - $6.96
		OR		
		Ceftriaxone IM	250 mg single dose	$3.95
		PLUS ONE of the following:		
		Azithromycin	1 g single dose	$5.23
		Doxycycline	100 mg BID for 7 days	7 days: $8.19
	SECOND LINE	**Ofloxacin**[4]	400 mg single dose **Not approved for children**	$1.53
		Ciprofloxacin[4]	500 mg single dose **Not approved for children < 18 years**	$0.70
		Spectinomycin IM[5]	2 g single dose	$14.77
		ANY ONE of the above PLUS ONE of the following:		
		Azithromycin	1 g single dose	$5.23
		Doxycycline	100 mg BID 7 days	7 days: $8.19
		Erythromycin[6]	2 g/day divided QID for 7 days. If not tolerated then 1 g/day divided QID for 14 days	7 days (2 g): $2.54

1) Must be reported to Medical Officer of Health. All sexual partners of patients with presumed sexually acquired urethritis should be evaluated and treated (CAN STI 2010; BASHH 2011). Repeat testing at 6 months is recommended.

2) It is recommended to routinely treat both *N. gonorrhoeae* and *C. trachomatis* concomitantly as these two pathogens often accompany each other. Where lab results are not available and there is urethral discharge, treat for both; if no urethral discharge is detected, defer antimicrobial treatment until results are available. Infections may be present without symptoms/signs or PMN response, but if present, treatment is required.

3) In pregnant and nursing mothers, the treatments of choice for gonococcal urethritis are cefixime, ceftriaxone, and spectinomycin. Azithromycin 1 g single dose or erythromycin (dose as above) should be used to treat concomitant chlamydial infection in pregnant and nursing women. Culture 4-5 days post treatment. Doxycycline and erythromycin estolate are contraindicated in pregnancy (MotheRisk 2008).

4) Ciprofloxacin can be considered if *Pseudomonas* is documented or suspected. Due to increased resistance, quinolones should only be considered as an alternative treatment option if susceptibility is demonstrated. Quinolones should not be used if there is a possibility the infection was acquired in places known to have increased resistance (e.g., South East Asia). If they are used in such cases, a test-of-cure is recommended.

5) If cefixime and spectinomycin is used, a test-of-cure is recommended. Spectinomycin is available through STI clinics.

6) If erythromycin is used, repeat testing after treatment is advised.

References: BASHH 2011; Bignell 2001; Brocklehurst 2007; CAN STI 2010; CDC 2010, 2012; Finnish Medical Society Duodecim 2006; Horner 2001; MotheRisk 2008; Smith 2007; Van Vranken 2007; Workowski 2006.

Modifying Circumstances	Probable Organism(s)	Antibiotic Choice(s)	Usual Dosage‡	Cost per Day

Urethritis – Gonococcal[1, 2]

Modifying Circumstances	Probable Organism(s)	Antibiotic Choice(s)	Usual Dosage‡	Cost per Day
CHILDREN < 9 YEARS	N. gonorrhoeae C. trachomatis[2]	FIRST LINE **Cefixime**[3]	8 mg/kg single dose (Maximum: 400 mg)	$0.19/kg
		OR		
		Ceftriaxone IM	125 mg single dose	$2.00
		ANY ONE of the above PLUS ONE of the following:		
		Azithromycin	10-15 mg/kg single dose (Maximum: 1 g)	$0.20 - $0.30/kg
		Erythromycin estolate[4]	40 mg/kg/day divided q6-8h for 7 days (Maximum: 500 mg QID)	7 days: $0.27/kg
		SECOND LINE **Spectinomycin IM**[5]	40 mg/kg/day divided q6-8h in a single dose (Maximum: 2 g)	2 g vial: $14.77
		PLUS ONE of the following:		
		Azithromycin	12-15 mg/kg single dose (Maximum: 1 g)	$0.20 - $0.30/kg
		Erythromycin estolate[4]	40 mg/kg/day divided q6-8h for 7 days (Maximum: 500 mg QID)	7 days: $0.27/kg

1) Must be reported to Medical Officer of Health.

2) It is recommended to routinely treat both N. gonorrhoeae and C. trachomatis concomitantly as these two pathogens often accompany each other. Where lab results are not available and there is urethral discharge, treat for both; if no urethral discharge is detected, defer antimicrobial treatment until results are available. Note that infections may be present without symptoms/signs or PMN response, but if present, treatment is required.

3) Antimicrobial susceptibility and follow-up culture should be performed if cefixime is used. If follow-up cannot be ensured, ceftriaxone IM should be used instead.

4) If erythromycin is used, repeat testing after treatment is advised.

5) If spectinomycin is used, a test-of-cure is recommended. Available through STI clinics.

References: BASHH 2011; Bignell 2001; CAN STI 2010; CDC 2010; Finnish Medical Society Duodecim 2006; Horner 2001; Workowski 2006.

© 2013 Anti-infective Review Panel

‡ Common oral dosage ranges are provided unless otherwise stated. Consult the drug monograph for details on age and condition-specific dosing.   **Page 85**

Modifying Circumstances	Probable Organism(s)		Antibiotic Choice(s)	Usual Dosage‡	Cost per Day

Urethritis - Nongonococcal [1, 2, 3]

Modifying Circumstances	Probable Organism(s)		Antibiotic Choice(s)	Usual Dosage‡	Cost per Day
ADOLESCENTS AND ADULTS ≥ 9 YEARS	C. trachomatis U. urealyticum M. genitalium	*FIRST LINE*	**Azithromycin**	1 g single dose	$5.23
			Doxycycline	100 mg BID for 7 days	7 days: $8.19
		SECOND LINE	**Erythromycin** [4]	2 g/day divided QID for 7 days. If not tolerated then 1 g/day divided QID for 14 days	7 days (2 g): $2.54
			Ofloxacin	300 mg BID for 7 days **Not approved for children < 18 years**	7 days: $21.45
CHILDREN < 9 YEARS		*FIRST LINE*	**Azithromycin**	10-15 mg/kg single dose (Maximum: 1 g)	$0.20 - $0.30/kg
			Erythromycin estolate [4]	40 mg/kg/day divided QID for 7 days (Maximum: 500 mg QID)	7 days: $0.27/kg

1) Must be reported to Medical Officer of Health. All sexual contacts with the patient during the 60 days preceding the onset of symptoms should be tested and empirically treated regardless of clinical findings and without waiting for test results (CAN STI 2010; CDC 2010). Resolution of symptoms can take up to 7 days after therapy has been completed. Test of cure not routinely recommended unless alternate regimen used, in children < 14 years, pregnancy or a non-genital site (e.g., eye) is involved.

2) In **pregnancy,** use azithromycin 1 g single dose or erythromycin (adult dosage as above). Alternative is amoxicillin 500 mg TID for 7 days. Erythromycin estolate is contraindicated.

3) Recurrent or persistent cases occur in 20-60% of men treated for acute nongonococcal urethritis. Ensure the patient was compliant with the initial regimen or the sex partner was treated. Consider other causes, such as *T. vaginalis*, tetracycline-resistant *U. urealyticum* or *N. gonorrhoeae*. If noncompliance or re-infection is ruled out, consider metronidazole 2 g in a single dose plus erythromycin 500 mg QID x 7 days OR azithromycin 1 g single dose (if not used for initial episode or compliance may be an issue).

4) If erythromycin is used, repeat testing after treatment is advised.

References: BASHH 2011; Bignell 2001; CAN STI 2010; CDC 2010; Finnish Medical Society Duodecim 2006; Horner 2001; Lanjouw 2009; Shahmanesh 2009; Smith 2007; Van Vranken 2007.

‡ Common oral dosage ranges are provided unless otherwise stated. Consult the drug monograph for details on age and condition-specific dosing.

Modifying Circumstances	Probable Organism(s)		Antibiotic Choice(s)	Usual Dosage‡	Cost per Day

Cervicitis [1, 2, 3, 4]

Modifying Circumstances	Probable Organism(s)		Antibiotic Choice(s)	Usual Dosage‡	Cost per Day
	C. trachomatis N. gonorrhoeae	**FIRST LINE**	**Cefixime**	400-800 mg single dose	$3.48 - $6.96
			PLUS ONE of the following:		
			Azithromycin	1 g in a single dose	$5.23
			Doxycycline	100 mg BID for 7 days	7 days: $8.19
		SECOND LINE	**Ofloxacin** [5]	400 mg single dose **Not approved for children**	$1.53
			Ciprofloxacin [5]	500 mg single dose **Not approved for children < 18 years**	$0.70
			Ceftriaxone IM	250 mg single dose	$3.95
			ONE of the above PLUS ONE of the following:		
			Azithromycin	1 g single dose	$5.23
			Doxycycline	100 mg BID for 7 days	7 days: $8.19
			Erythromycin [6]	2 g/day divided QID for 7 days. If not tolerated then 1 g/day divided QID for 14 days	7 days (2 g): $2.54

1) Must be reported to Medical Officer of Health. All sex partners should be evaluated if they had sexual contact with the patient during the 60 days preceding the onset of symptoms (CDC 2010).

2) The criteria for defining cervicitis, especially when signs are minimal, are not well standardized. Generally, an inflammation of the cervix with a mucopurulent or purulent cervical discharge and an increased number of polymorphonuclear leucocytes. Cervicitis does not occur in prepubertal girls; the counterpart is prepubertal vaginitis. Cervicitis and vaginitis frequently coexist, therefore patients should be evaluated for both.

3) Defer treatment until microbiological results are available in "at-risk" patients including sexually active women, where no mucopurulent or purulent endocervical discharge and no gram-negative intracellular diplococci are present.

4) **Pregnancy:** use cefixime, ceftriaxone or spectinomycin. If allergic to penicillins, then azithromycin or erythromycin can be used instead. Erythromycin estolate is contraindicated in pregnancy.

5) Ciprofloxacin can be considered if *Pseudomonas* is documented or suspected. Due to increased resistance, quinolones should only be considered as an alternative treatment option if susceptibility is demonstrated. Quinolones should not be used if there is a possibility the infection was acquired in places known to have increased resistance (e.g., South East Asia). If they are used in such cases, a test-of-cure is recommended.

6) If erythromycin is used, repeat testing after treatment is advised.

References: CAN STI 2010; CDC 2010; Chandran 2004; Finnish Medical Society Duodecim 2006; Lusk 2008; Smith 2007; Workowski 2006.

© 2013 Anti-infective Review Panel

‡ Common oral dosage ranges are provided unless otherwise stated. Consult the drug monograph for details on age and condition-specific dosing. **Page 87**

Modifying Circumstances	Probable Organism(s)	Antibiotic Choice(s)		Usual Dosage‡	Cost per Day

Herpes Simplex Virus – Adult, Genital Herpes [1, 2] (Normal Host)

Modifying Circumstances	Probable Organism(s)	Antibiotic Choice(s)		Usual Dosage‡	Cost per Day
FIRST SYMPTOMATIC EPISODE [3, 4]	Herpes Simplex type 1 or 2	*FIRST LINE*	Acyclovir	400 mg TID for 5 to 7 days	$1.90
			Famciclovir	250 mg TID for 5 to 7 days	$2.54
			Valacyclovir	500-1000 mg BID for 5 to 7 days	$1.70 - $3.39
ACUTE RECURRENT ≤ 6 EPISODES PER YEAR [4]		*FIRST LINE*	Acyclovir	400 mg TID for 5 days or 800 mg BID for 5 days or 800 mg TID for 2 days	$1.90 - $3.80
			Famciclovir	125 mg BID for 5 days	$4.00
			Valacyclovir	500 mg BID for 3 days or 1000 mg once daily for 3 days	$1.70
CHRONIC SUPPRESSIVE > 6 EPISODES PER YEAR [5] (NON-PREGNANT)		*FIRST LINE*	Acyclovir	400 mg BID	$1.27
			Famciclovir	250 mg BID	$1.69
			Valacyclovir [6]	250 mg BID or 500 mg daily If > 9 episodes per year then 1000 mg daily	$0.85

(Pregnancy) [7]

Modifying Circumstances	Probable Organism(s)	Antibiotic Choice(s)		Usual Dosage‡	Cost per Day
FIRST SYMPTOMATIC EPISODE [3, 4]	Herpes Simplex type 1 or 2	*FIRST LINE*	Acyclovir	200 mg 5 times daily for 5 to 10 days	$4.28
PRIOR INFECTION WITHIN PREVIOUS YEAR	Prophylaxis at 36 weeks		Acyclovir	200 mg QID or 400 mg TID	$4.28
			Valacyclovir	500 mg BID	$1.70

(Immunocompromised Host)

More likely to require more aggressive therapies (i.e., IV 5-10 mg/kg q8h x 5-10 days or high dose oral therapy). Consultation with a colleague experienced in this area should be sought.

Continued ...

© 2013 Anti-infective Review Panel
Page 88   ‡ Common oral dosage ranges are provided unless otherwise stated. Consult the drug monograph for details on age and condition-specific dosing.

Herpes Simplex Virus – Adult, Genital Herpes (Normal Host)

1) Patients should be advised to abstain from sexual activity when lesions or prodromal symptoms are present and are encouraged to inform their sex partners that they have genital herpes. Sexual transmission of herpes simplex virus (HSV) may occur during asymptomatic periods where there is no evidence of lesions. The use of condoms during all sexual exposures with new sex partners should also be encouraged, although condoms may not be effective in preventing transmission of HSV because of location of lesions or asymptomatic shedding.

2) Initiate therapy within 72 hours of onset of signs and symptoms for most benefit. Topical antivirals offer minimal clinical benefit and their use is not recommended. Counseling on natural history of disease, asymptomatic shedding, sexual and perinatal transmission, and methods to reduce transmission, should be an integral component of clinical management. **Initiation of therapy within one day of lesion onset or during prodrome that precedes outbreaks, is encouraged to ensure effective treatment of recurrent herpes. Patients can be provided with a supply of medication or a prescription so that self-initiation of treatment can occur immediately when symptoms begin** (CDC 2010).

3) Primary infections are frequently asymptomatic. The 'first' episode here includes symptomatic primary and non-primary first episodes. A primary episode is the first clinically evident episode in a seronegative patient; usual incubation for symptomatic primary infection is 2 to 21 days. Non-primary is first clinically evident episode in a seropositive patient; short or long incubation (sometimes years), systemic symptoms unusual.

4) No role for topical antivirals. Analgesics and laxatives may be required. There may be a small clinical advantage to using famciclovir or valacyclovir over acyclovir for episodic therapy.

5) The frequency of recurrent genital herpes is reduced by 70-80% with suppressive therapy in those individuals who experience ≥ 6 recurrences per year (CDC 2010). Usual duration of therapy is 3-6 months. The objectives of chronic suppressive treatment include reduction of frequency and severity of recurrences, reduction of asymptomatic HSV shedding, and psychological benefit to the patient. Some patients may require higher doses or greater dosing frequency. Reassess therapy every 6-12 months since frequency of recurrent outbreaks diminishes over time in many patients (CDC 2010). Some experts recommend discontinuing suppressive therapy after one year to reassess recurrence frequency (Patel 2001).

6) Valacyclovir 1000 mg daily appears to be more effective than valacyclovir 500 mg daily in patients who have very frequent recurrences of > 9 episodes per year (Reitano 1998).

7) A primary outbreak in the first trimester constitutes a higher risk for perinatal transmission than does recurrent infection and warrants treatment. The risk of vertical transmission when a primary outbreak occurs at the time of delivery is approximately 30-60%; consider cesarean delivery if infection is late in the third trimester. For women with prior infection within the previous year, prophylaxis at 36 weeks gestation is recommended (CAN STI 2010; CDC 2010; Scott 2002; Sheffield 2006; SOGC 2008; Watts 2003).

References: Aoki 2006; Barton 2007; BASHH 2008; Brady 2004; CAN STI 2010; CDC 2010; Gupta 2007; Leone 2002; Patel 2005; Prodigy 2003; Reitano 1998; Scott 2002; Sen 2007; Sheffield 2006; SOGC 2008; Wald 2002; Watts 2003.

Modifying Circumstances	Probable Organism(s)	Antibiotic Choice(s)	Usual Dosage‡	Cost per Day

Herpes Simplex Virus – Children, Genital Herpes [1, 2]
(Normal Host)

Modifying Circumstances	Probable Organism(s)	Antibiotic Choice(s)	Usual Dosage‡	Cost per Day
FIRST SYMPTOMATIC EPISODE [3]	Herpes Simplex type 1 or 2	Acyclovir	No data to indicate if treatment is effective when rash present longer than 72 hours. 20 mg/kg/day (Maximum: 200 mg) QID for 5 to 7 days Severe may require IV 500-750 mg/m^2 q8h x 7 days	$0.44/kg
ACUTE RECURRENCE		No data to support use of acyclovir, although efficacy and safety are probably not different than for adults.		
CHRONIC SUPPRESSIVE		No data available.		

(Immunocompromised Host)

More likely to require more aggressive therapies (i.e., IV or high-dose oral therapy)

Consultation with a colleague experienced in this area should be sought.

1) Initiate therapy within 72 hours of onset of signs and symptoms for most benefit.

2) **When a child > 3 months of age presents with a case of genital or perianal herpes, one should consider whether sexual abuse is involved. If sexual abuse is suspected, investigate the possibility of other sexually transmitted diseases. Suspected or known sexual abuse of a child must be reported by the primary health care provider to the local agency responsible for child protection.**

3) The 'first' episode here includes symptomatic primary and nonprimary first episodes. A primary episode is the first clinically evident episode in a seronegative patient; usual incubation for symptomatic primary infection is 2 to 21 days. Non-primary is first clinically evident episode in a seropositive patient; short or long incubation (sometimes years), systemic symptoms unusual.

References: Aoki 2006; Brady 2004; CAN STI 2010; CDC 2010; Jones 2004; Leone 2002; Patel 2001; Reitano 1998.

Modifying Circumstances	Probable Organism(s)	Antibiotic Choice(s)	Usual Dosage‡	Cost per Day

External Genital Warts (EGW) – Adult [1, 2, 3]

		Patient-applied immunomodulating treatment [4]		
	Human Papilloma Virus (HPV, usually types 6 & 11)	**Imiquimod 5% cream (one single-use sachet covers ~20 cm² or ~palm of a hand)**	Apply at bedtime three times per week for up to 16 weeks. Wash off 6-10 hours after application with soap & water.	3 pkgs (~1 week): $34.26
		Patient-applied caustic treatment [4, 5]		
EXTERNAL GENITAL AND PERIANAL WARTS		**Podofilox (podophyllotoxin) 0.5% solution**	1 treatment cycle: Apply BID in morning and at bedtime (or q12h) for 3 days, followed by no therapy for 4 days.	Condyline 3.5 mL: $39.04 Wartec 3 mL: $40.47
		Total area treated should be ≤ 10cm²; total volume used ≤ 0.5 mL/day	Repeat if necessary up to a maximum of 4 cycles. Where possible a health care provider should apply the initial treatment to demonstrate technique.	
		Physician-administered treatment [5]		
		Cryotherapy [6]	Repeat application of liquid nitrogen or cryoprobe every 1-2 weeks (for maximum 8 weeks)	
		Podophyllin resin 10-25 % in compound tincture of benzoin [7] **Total area treated should be ≤ 10cm²; total volume used ≤ 0.5 mL/day**	Apply a small amount to warts, allow to dry. If necessary, treatment can be repeated weekly. Some specialists suggest washing off resin 1-4 hours after application.	25 mL: $22.55
		Trichloroacetic acid [8] **(TCA) 80-90% in 70% ethyl alcohol**	Apply a small amount to warts, allow to dry and form a white frosting. If necessary, treatment can be repeated weekly. To prevent burning discomfort, apply 5% EMLA cream around warts to be treated, 10-20 minutes prior to therapy.	
		Laser therapy	Repeat laser vaporization is optional.	
		Surgical removal	Tangential scissor excision, tangential shave excision, curettage, or electrosurgery (fulguration/excision)	

Continued ...

Modifying Circumstances	Probable Organism(s)	Antibiotic Choice(s)	Usual Dosage‡	Cost per Day

External Genital Warts (EGW) – Adult [1, 2, 3]

MORE EXTENSIVE OR RESISTANT EXTERNAL GENITAL AND PERIANAL WARTS[9]		Refer to Specialist for: Electrosurgery Laser surgery Loop Electro-surgical Excision Procedure (LEEP)		

1) Most patients have ≤ 10 genital warts, with a total wart area of 0.5-1.0 cm. The wart should be confirmed by biopsy if diagnosis is uncertain, lesions are non-responsive or worsen under treatment, the patient is immunocompromised (more likely to have dysplasia, poor response, relapse) or the wart is pigmented, indurated, fixed and/or ulcerated (CDC 2010). The main treatment objective is to remove symptomatic warts, eradicate the infection, prevent long-term sequelae and possibly interrupt HPV transmission. No one treatment is ideal for all warts or all patients and should be selected based on several factors including wart size, location, number, morphology, patient preference, provider experience, cost, convenience and adverse effects. It is important to note that deciding not to treat is an option at any site as warts resolve spontaneously in some patients (20% do so within 6 months) (PAB 2002; Von Krogh 2000; Zanotti 2002).

2) Warts respond to most treatment modalities with those located on moist surfaces and/or intertriginous areas responding better to topical treatment than warts on drier surfaces (CDC 2010). Soft, non-keratinised warts respond well to podophyllotoxin and TCA. Keratinised lesions are better treated with physical ablative methods, such as cryotherapy, excision or electrocautery. Imiquimod may be suitable for both types (Maw 2002). If no significant response is seen within 4-6 weeks of treatment (except imiquimod), consider changing treatment or referral.

3) Genital warts can proliferate and become friable during pregnancy and many specialists recommend removing them in pregnant women (CDC 2010). Podophyllotoxin and podophyllin should not be used in pregnancy. There are no adequate and controlled clinical studies of imiquimod cream in pregnant women thus potential benefits must be weighed against potential risks.

4) For successful and safe use of patient-applied therapies, the patient must be able to see, recognize and reach their warts, and be able to follow application instructions successfully (PAB 2002). It has been suggested that treatment for lesions each measuring > 4 cm^2 should take place under direct medical supervision (Maw 2002).

5) These therapeutic modalities do not address the issue of subclinical (aceto-white) HPV infection. Including imiquimod cream as an adjunct (either pre or post-therapy) may reduce the high recurrence rates seen when treatments are used as monotherapy (Heinzerling 2003; Hoyme 2002).

6) Cryotherapy is effective for both dry and moist, external and internal warts (PAB 2002). Freezing is usually continued until a frozen area slightly larger (1-2 mm) than the diameter of the wart is formed (Maw 2002; Beutner 1997). Refer to a specialist for more focused freezing using fine probes on nitrous oxide or carbon dioxide cryoguns (PAB 2002). Injected local or topical anesthetic is not required, but can reduce discomfort due to cryotherapy (Beutner 1998), especially if warts are present in many areas or a large area (CDC 2010).

7) Podophyllin is available in Canada but has more adverse affects and inferior efficacy to podophyllotoxin and has been associated with severe local reactions and systemic effects. It should be avoided on the cervix, in the anal canal and during pregnancy (Maw 2002).

8) If an excess amount of TCA is applied, the treated area should be powdered with talc, sodium bicarbonate or liquid soap to remove the unreacted acid (CDC 2010). TCA is not recommended for large-volume warts and the surrounding area should be protected with petroleum jelly (Maw 2002). Apply sparingly and allow to dry before the patient sits or stands to prevent spread to normal tissues (PAB 2002).

9) Refer to specialist in cases of large volume disseminated disease, including extensive genital, urethral meatal or anal warts, intraepithelial neoplasia, immunosuppressed patients or in children.

References: Arany 1999; BASHH 2008; Beutner 1997, 1998; Birley 2001; CAN STI 2010; CDC 2010; Edwards 1998; Einarson 2006; Heinzerling 2003; Hoyme 2002; Langley 1999; LCDC 1998; Maw 2000, 2002; Moore 2001; O'Mahoney 2005; PAB 2002; Reese 2000; Roy 1997; Tyring 1998; Von Krogh 2000, 2001; Wiley 2002, 2003; Zanotti 2002.

© 2013 Anti-infective Review Panel

Page 92   ‡ Common oral dosage ranges are provided unless otherwise stated. Consult the drug monograph for details on age and condition-specific dosing.

Central Nervous System Infections

Modifying Circumstances	Probable Organism(s)		Antibiotic Choice(s)	Usual Dosage‡	Cost per Day

Bacterial Meningitis – Adult [1, 2, 3, 4]

Modifying Circumstances	Probable Organism(s)		Antibiotic Choice(s)	Usual Dosage‡	Cost per Day
18-50 YEARS	S. pneumoniae N. meningitidis H. influenzae type B	FIRST LINE	[Ceftriaxone IV	2 g q12h for first 48 hours then q24h	$24.14
			OR		
			Cefotaxime IV]	2 g q6h	$73.60
			+/-		
			Ampicillin IV [5] +/-	2 g q4-6h	$21.20 - $31.80
			Vancomycin IV [2]	500 mg q6h or 1 g q12h (Individualize dosing)	1 g: $15.50
> 50 YEARS (Includes adults with alcoholism and/or other debilitating illness)	S. pneumoniae Listeria monocytogenes Enteric Gram -ve N. meningitidis	FIRST LINE	[Cefotaxime IV	2 g q4-6h	$73.60
			OR		
			Ceftriaxone IV]	2 g q12h for first 48 hours then q24h	$24.14
			PLUS		
			Ampicillin IV [5] +/-	2 g q4-6h	$21.20 - $31.80
			Vancomycin IV [2]	500 mg q6h or 1 g q12h (Individualize dosing)	1 g: $15.50
		SECOND LINE	TMP/SMX IV	160-240 mg q6-12h (Trimethoprim component)	5 mL vial: $5.75

© 2013 Anti-infective Review Panel

TMP/SMX = Trimethoprim / Sulfamethoxazole

Page 94   ‡ Common oral dosage ranges are provided unless otherwise stated. Consult the drug monograph for details on age and condition-specific dosing.

Bacterial Meningitis – Adult

1) Reportable to Medical Officer of Health. Contact Public Health regarding post-exposure prophylaxis for close contacts with antibiotics and/or vaccines.
The following is a guide (Cha'vez-Bueno 2005; El Bashir 2003; PHAC 2005, 2009; UK 2012):

   H. influenzae type b infection:
   - All home contacts (except those that are completely immunized against Hib) should be given rifampin 20 mg/kg/day (maximum 600 mg/day) for 4 days.
   - All children who are less than 5 years of age and who are unvaccinated or incompletely vaccinated should be brought up to date by administration of the recommended doses of a licensed Hib conjugate vaccine.

   Meningococcal infection - Chemoprophylaxis for Close Contacts (give one of the following):
   - Ciprofloxacin: Adult: 500 mg PO single dose. Children/adolescents as necessary: 10 mg/kg (not to exceed a maximum of 500 mg).
   - Rifampin: Adult: 600 mg q12h x 4 doses. Children > 1 month: 10 mg/kg (Maximum: 600 mg) per dose q12h x 4 doses; infants < 1 month: 5 mg/kg per dose q12h x 4 doses orally.
   - Ceftriaxone: Adults: 250 mg IM x 1 dose. Children < 12 years: 125 mg IM x 1 dose.
   - Unvaccinated children and close contacts aged > 2 years (with possible continuing exposure to the *N. meningitides* strain which has caused a case of meningitis) should be offered conjugate group C meningococcal vaccine, if the infection is type C, or quadrivalent vaccine, if the infection is type A, Y or W135.
   - Consider chemoprophylaxis for index patients before hospital discharge unless they have been treated with ceftriaxone (known to eradicate carriage) (Purcell 2004).

   Pneumococcal meningitis:
   - Chemoprophylaxis not indicated.

   Other types of bacterial meningitis:
   - Chemoprophylaxis not indicated.

2) **Initial empiric therapy should be a 3rd generation cephalosporin (ceftriaxone or cefotaxime) until the pathogen is identified and antibiotic susceptibility determined. If penicillin-resistant pneumococcus is a possibility, then add vancomycin. Discontinue vancomycin as soon as 3rd-generation cephalosporin resistance is excluded.** In cases of penicillin allergy, cefotaxime or ceftriaxone can be used (see page viii for more information). Chloramphenicol monotherapy has failed against drug resistant *S. pneumoniae* but can be added where there is a severe ß-lactam allergy to cover for meningococcus.

3) The optimal duration of treatment is uncertain. The following is a general guide (Quagliarello 1997):

   Meningococcal: 7-10 days

   H. influenzae: 7-10 days

   S. pneumoniae: 10-14 days

   Other (such as *L. monocytogenes*, *S. agalactiae*, gram-negative bacilli other than *H. influenzae*): 14-28 days

4) Dexamethasone 10 mg IV every 6 hours for 4 days has been shown to decrease mortality in patients with *S. pneumoniae* meningitis with no significant increase in side effects. The benefit is less clear in patients with meningococcal meningitis. Dexamethasone should be initiated 15-20 minutes prior to or concurrently with the first dose of antibiotic (Chaudhuri 2004; de Gans 2002; van de Beek 2007).

5) *Listeria monocytogenes* requires ampicillin to be added.

References: Band 1984; CAN 2006; CDC 2013; Chaudhuri 2004, 2008; Cha'vez-Bueno 2005; de Gans 2002; El Bashir 2003; Gardner 2006; Kim 2010; Moyneux 2011; NACI 2009; PHAC 2005, 2009, 2012; Purcell 2004; Quagliarello 1997; Tunkel 2004; van de Beek 2006, 2007; UK 2012.

Modifying Circumstances	Probable Organism(s)		Antibiotic Choice(s)	Usual Dosage‡	Cost per Day

Bacterial Meningitis – Children [1, 2, 3]

Modifying Circumstances	Probable Organism(s)		Antibiotic Choice(s)	Usual Dosage‡	Cost per Day
INFANTS 1 - 3 MONTHS	Group B Strep E. coli Listeria[5] monocytogenes S. pneumoniae N. meningitidis H. influenzae type B	FIRST LINE	[Cefotaxime IV [4]	200 mg/kg/day divided q6-8h (Maximum: 8 g/day)	$1.84/kg
			OR		
			Ceftriaxone IV [4]]	80-100 mg/kg/day divided q12h for first 2 days then q24h (Maximum: 4 g/day)	$1.26 - $1.58/kg
			ONE of the above PLUS:		
			Ampicillin IV [5]	200-400 mg/kg/day divided q4-6h (Maximum: 10 g/day)	$0.05 - $0.08/kg
CHILDREN AND YOUNG ADULT 3 MONTHS TO 18 YEARS	S. pneumoniae N. meningitidis H. influenzae type B	FIRST LINE	[Cefotaxime IV [4]	200-300 mg/kg/day divided q6-8h (Maximum: 8 g/day)	$1.84/kg
			OR		
			Ceftriaxone IV [4]]	80-100 mg/kg/day divided q12h for first 2 days then q24h (Maximum: 4 g/day)	$1.30 - $1.70/kg
			PLUS		
			Vancomycin IV [2]	10-15 mg/kg per dose q6h (Maximum: 2 g/day) (Individualize dosing)	$2.92 - $4.39/kg

Continued ...

© 2013 Anti-infective Review Panel

Page 96   ‡ Common oral dosage ranges are provided unless otherwise stated. Consult the drug monograph for details on age and condition-specific dosing.

Bacterial Meningitis – Children

1) Reportable to Medical Officer of Health. Contact Public Health regarding post-exposure prophylaxis for close contacts with antibiotics and/or vaccines.
   The following is a guide (Cha'vez-Bueno 2005; El Bashir 2003; PHAC 2005, 2009; UK 2012):

   H. influenzae type b infection:
   - All home contacts (except those that are completely immunized against Hib) should be given rifampin 20 mg/kg/day (maximum 600 mg/day) for 4 days.
   - All children who are less than 5 years of age and who are unvaccinated or incompletely vaccinated should be brought up to date by administration of the recommended doses of a licensed Hib conjugate vaccine.

   Meningococcal infection - Chemoprophylaxis for Close Contacts (give one of the following):
   - Ciprofloxacin: Adult: 500 mg PO single dose. Children/adolescents as necessary: 10 mg/kg (not to exceed a maximum of 500 mg).
   - Rifampin: Adult: 600 mg q12h x 4 doses. Children > 1 month: 10 mg/kg (Maximum: 600 mg) per dose q12h x 4 doses; infants < 1 month: 5 mg/kg per dose q12h x 4 doses orally.
   - Ceftriaxone: Adults: 250 mg IM x 1 dose. Children < 12 years: 125 mg IM x 1 dose.
   - Unvaccinated children and close contacts aged > 2 years (with possible continuing exposure to the *N. meningitides* strain which has caused a case of meningitis) should be offered conjugate group C meningococcal vaccine, if the infection is type C, or quadrivalent vaccine, if the infection is type A, Y, or W135.
   - Consider chemoprophylaxis for index patients before hospital discharge unless they have been treated with ceftriaxone (known to eradicate carriage) (Purcell 2004).

   Pneumococcal meningitis:
   - Chemoprophylaxis not indicated.

   Other types of bacterial meningitis:
   - Chemoprophylaxis not indicated.

2) Initial empiric treatment of bacterial meningitis in infants six weeks of age and older consists of a combination of a 3rd-generation cephalosporin and vancomycin (aiming for a peak serum vancomycin level of 30 to 40 mg/L and a trough level of 5 to 10 mg/L daily). Rifampin has been proposed as an alternative to the cephalosporins. Definitive therapy and the duration of therapy should be guided by susceptibility results of the organism identified. **Vancomycin should be discontinued as soon as 3rd generation cephalosporin resistance is excluded** (Can Paed Soc 2012). In cases of penicillin allergy, cefotaxime or ceftriaxone can be used (see page viii for more information).

3) Dexamethasone (0.6 mg/kg/day IV divided q6h for 4 days or 0.8 mg/kg/day divided q12h for 2 to 4 days) as an adjunct to antibiotic therapy decreases the risk of severe hearing loss in both *H. influenzae* and non-*H. influenzae* meningitis. The first dose should be given 15-20 minutes prior to or concurrently with the first dose of antibiotic. Due to the lack of data, dexamethasone is not recommended in neonates (Saez-Llorens 2003; van de Beek 2007).

4) Ceftriaxone safety is not yet established in neonates and is therefore only recommended after 1 month of age. Cefotaxime is approved from day 0 of life: In neonates, a dosage of 100 mg/kg/day divided q12h from 0-1 week and 150 mg/kg/day divided q8h from 1-4 weeks is recommended. If weight is over 50 kg, use adult dosage.

5) *Listeria monocytogenes* requires ampicillin to be added

References: AAP 2006; Band 1984; Bilukha 2005; CAN 2006; Can Paed Soc 2012; CDC 2013; Chaudhuri 2004, 2008; Cha'vez-Bueno 2005; El Bashir 2003; Kim 2010; Moyneux 2011; NACI 2009; NICE 2010; PHAC 2005, 2009, 2012; Purcell 2004; Quagliarello 1997; Roine 2000; Saez-Llorens 2003; SIGN 2008; Singhi 2002; Tunkel 2004; van de Beek 2007; UK 2012.

Gastrointestinal Infections

H. pylori (Helicobacter pylori) Infection [1, 2, 3]

FIRST-LINE COMBINATIONS [4]	DURATION OF THERAPY
(Lansoprazole 30 mg [5] or Omeprazole 20 mg or Pantoprazole 40 mg or Rabeprazole 20 mg or Esomeprazole 20 mg) = **PPI (proton pump inhibitor)** BID Amoxicillin 1000 mg BID Clarithromycin 500 mg BID	ONE week
OR	
PPI BID Metronidazole [6] 500 mg BID Clarithromycin 500 mg or 250 mg BID	ONE week
SECOND-LINE COMBINATIONS	
PPI BID Metronidazole [6] 500 mg BID Amoxicillin 1000 mg BID	ONE week
OR	
PPI BID Bismuth Subsalicylate [3] 2 tabs or 30 mL QID Metronidazole [6] 250 mg QID Tetracycline 500 mg QID	7-14 days

Continued ...

H. pylori (Helicobacter pylori) Infection

1) **Who to treat:** Treat all *H. pylori* positive patients with unequivocal duodenal or gastric ulcers, active or inactive. Even if an NSAID is the suspected etiological agent, eradicating the documented *H. pylori* infection is appropriate. A test-and-treat strategy is recommended for patients with uninvestigated dyspepsia who are under the age of 55 years and have no "alarm features" (bleeding, anemia, early satiety, unexplained weight loss, progressive dysphagia, odynophagia, recurrent vomiting, family history of GI cancer, previous esophagogastric malignancy). Patients with gastric MALToma who are *H. pylori* positive, should be treated.

   Diagnosis: The non-invasive urea breath test should be used for routine diagnosis unless endoscopy is indicated for another reason. The accuracy of serology is associated with more variability among laboratories. Serology has a higher rate of false-positive results in young patients, in whom the prevalence of infection is lower. Invasive tests require endoscopy but are definitive.

   Follow-up: Confirmation of eradication is suggested for complicated (bleeding, perforation, stricture) or refractory ulcers, but is controversial after the medical management of uncomplicated ulcers in patients who remain asymptomatic. Follow-up testing should be done no earlier than one month after stopping agents capable of suppressing *H. pylori* (i.e., antimicrobials, PPIs, H_2 receptor antagonists, bismuth containing compounds). Serology is not recommended for confirming eradication of infection because antibodies may persist for many months after eradication (McColl 2010). To minimize the risk of recurrences, patients should be advised to stop NSAID use, stop smoking and minimize the use of alcohol.

2) Bacterial resistance has been reported to metronidazole and clarithromycin but rarely to amoxicillin and none to tetracycline. Treatment failure options include a subsequent trial using an alternative antibiotic. For example, if failure occurred with amoxicillin, then a metronidazole combination could be considered. Note that treatment failure is often due to non-compliance. The following alternative 10-day regimen can be considered in patients that have failed 1st and 2nd-line treatment. This regimen should not be overused due to concerns of resistance (Chey 2007; Gisbert 2006):

   PPI BID

   Amoxicillin 1 g BID

   Levofloxacin 500 mg OD

3) Avoid bismuth subsalicylate and antacids if severe renal impairment present (creatinine clearance < 30 mL/min). Substitute ranitidine 150 mg BID if PPI intolerant.

4) In patients older than 55 years with no history of peptic ulcer disease, a 5-day course of treatment with the following quadruple therapy combination may be considered. An open-label RCT found that this combination is associated with an ~ 89% eradication rate (Treiber 2002):

   Ranitidine 300 mg BID or Lansoprazole 30 mg BID plus

   Amoxicillin 1 g BID plus

   Clarithromycin 250 mg BID plus

   Metronidazole 500 mg BID

5) A combination therapy of lansoprazole, amoxicillin and clarithromycin is available in a daily administration blister pack (i.e., Hp-PAC).

6) Advise patient NOT to take any alcoholic beverages during metronidazole therapy and for 48 hours post-treatment to prevent disulfiram-like reaction.

References: Abu-Mahfouz 1997; Chey 2007; Egan 2007; Ford 2006; Gisbert 2006; Gold 2000; Hunt 1998, 1999, 2004; Jones 2005; ICSI 2006; Laine 2003; Leal-Herrera 2003; Malfertheiner 2007; McColl 2010; Perri 2001; Sander 2000; Sebastian 2002; Selgrad 2009; SIGN 2008; Treiber 2002; Vaira 2007; Veldhuyzen va Zanten 2000; Vergara 2003; Zagari 2007.

Modifying Circumstances	Probable Organism(s)		Antibiotic Choice(s)	Usual Dosage‡	Cost per Day

Traveller's Diarrhea – Treatment and Prevention [1,2,3,4]

Modifying Circumstances	Probable Organism(s)		Antibiotic Choice(s)	Usual Dosage‡	Cost per Day
MILD TO MODERATE DIARRHEA (Up to 3 movements per day; no blood or fever)	Enterotoxigenic *E.coli (ETEC)* *Campylobacter* *Salmonella* *Shigella* *Viruses* *Protozoa*	*FIRST LINE*	Loperamide	4 mg STAT, then 2 mg after each loose stool (Maximum: 8 doses/day)	**Over-the-counter agent**
			Bismuth subsalicylate (Pepto Bismol)	2 tabs or 30 mL, repeat q30 minutes as needed (Maximum: 8 doses/day) **(Prevention: 2 tabs or 30 mL QID with meals and in evening)**	**Over-the-counter-agent**
MODERATE (3-5 movements per day; no blood or fever) **TO** **SEVERE** [5] (blood and/or fever)		*FIRST LINE*	Ofloxacin [6]	400 mg single dose or 300 mg BID for 3 days **(Prevention: 300 mg daily)**	$1.53 3 day: $9.19
			Norfloxacin [6]	800 mg single dose or 400 mg BID for 1-3 days **(Prevention: 400 mg daily)**	$2.18 3 day: $6.54
			Ciprofloxacin [6]	750 mg single dose or 500 mg BID for 1-3 days **(Prevention: 500 mg daily)**	$1.28 3 day: $4.20
			Levofloxacin [6]	500 mg daily for 1-3 days **(Prevention: 500 mg daily)**	$1.37 3 day: $4.11
			Azithromycin [7]	1000 mg single dose or 500 mg daily for 1-3 days **Children:** 10 mg/kg/day for 3 days	$5.23 3 day: $7.83 $0.20/kg

Traveller's Diarrhea – Treatment and Prevention

1) **Prevention:** Boil it, cook it, peel it, or forget it. Avoid raw or undercook meats, fish and seafood; unpasteurized dairy products; tap water and ice cubes; cold sauces and toppings; ground-grown leafy greens, vegetables, and fruits washed in untreated water, food from street vendors unless served piping hot (Green 2011; Hill 2010).
   Mild traveller's diarrhea will usually resolve in 24 hours with anti-motility agents and fluids. Symptoms persisting more than 2 weeks after returning home should be investigated thoroughly. Prophylaxis should **only** be used in patients at risk of the complications of diarrheal illness. Drugs taken for prevention should be started on the first day in the area of risk and continued for 1 or 2 days after returning home, to a maximum of 3 weeks total. If possible, one dose can be given initially and patient response evaluated over the following 12-24 hours. If diarrhea is improved, then the antibiotic can be discontinued, otherwise therapy can be continued for up to 3 days. Consult product monographs for children's dosing.

2) **Maintenance of fluid balance is vital**. Clear fluid diet of carbonated beverages, fruit juices, hot tea or purified water and salted crackers. Moderate diarrhea may benefit from electrolyte-containing solutions. Severe diarrhea, particularly in young children, requires careful fluid replacement with a solution of 3.5 g sodium chloride, 2.5 g sodium bicarbonate, 1.5 g potassium chloride and 20 g of glucose in 1 L of safe water or commercial preparations (Pedialyte, Gastrolyte) can be used.

3) While preliminary evidence suggests that probiotics, such as *Lactobacillus GG* and *Saccharomyces boulardii* may be effective in preventing traveller's diarrhea (DuPont 2006; McFarland 2005) further research is required before they can be definitively recommended (CDC Yellow Book 2008; Guandalini 2011; IDSA 2006; Ritchie 2012; Sazawal 2006).

4) The use of an oral, inactivated traveller's diarrhea and cholera vaccine (e.g., Dukoral™) as a prevention strategy for traveller's diarrhea is of limited value and cannot be routinely recommended for the majority of travellers. The vaccine may be considered for selected high-risk, short-term travellers, including young children aged > 2 years, patients with chronic illness, those with increased risk of acquiring traveller's diarrhea, such as gastric hypochlorhydria, immunocompromised, history of repeated severe traveller's diarrhea or those for who a brief illness cannot be tolerated (CCDR 2005; Jelinek 2008; NACI 2006).

5) Avoid anti-motility agents in high fever and bloody diarrhea since the agents have been shown to prolong invasive infection with *Shigella, Salmonella* and *Campylobacter*. Antimotility agents should be used in combination with antibiotics; avoid their use in children < 3 years old. TMP/SMX could be considered an alternative option, although substantial resistance has been documented globally and it is ineffective against *Campylobacter* and should only be used in areas with low rates of this infection (e.g., central Mexico).

6) For children less than 16 years old, fluoroquinolones are generally not recommended; however, for moderate to severe traveller's diarrhea a short course (1-3 days) may be considered as an alternative for children intolerant or allergic to azithromycin. Ciprofloxacin 15-20 mg/kg (Maximum: 500mg) q12h for 3 days is suggested (CCDR 2010; Plourde 2003).

7) Azithromycin is recommended primarily for Thailand, India, Nepal and Indonesia where *Campylobacter* resistance to quinolones is high. Azithromycin is considered the drug of choice for children because of safety, tolerability and ease of administration. It may be used as a prophylactic agent in select children at high risk and for treatment of children with moderate to severe diarrhea (Ang 2008; Plourde 2003).

References: Adachi 2003; Ang 2008; Casburn-Jones 2004; CCDR 2005, 2010; CDC Yellow Book 2008; Cook 1999; DuPont 2006, 2008, 2009; Green 2011; Guandalini 2011; Guerrant 2001; Hill 2006, 2008, 2010; Jelinek 2008; McFarland 2005; Medical Letter 2008; MetroDis 2003; Plourde 2003; Ritchie 2012; Ruddock 2004; Sazawal 2006; Tham 2010; Thielman 2004; WHO 2004.

Modifying Circumstances	Probable Organism(s)		Antibiotic Choice(s)	Usual Dosage‡	Cost per Day

C. difficile Infection (CDI) [1, 2]

Modifying Circumstances	Probable Organism(s)		Antibiotic Choice(s)	Usual Dosage‡	Cost per Day
ADULTS AND CHILDREN MILD-MODERATE $WBC < 15 \times 10^9/L$ and SCr < 1.5 x baseline	C. difficile	**FIRST LINE**	Metronidazole - ORAL	500 mg TID or 250 mg QID (if 500 mg not tolerated) for 10-14 days **Children:** 15-30 mg/kg/day orally divided TID-QID (Maximum: 2 g/day)	$0.24 - $0.38 $0.02 - $0.04/kg
SEVERE $WBC \geq 15 \times 10^9/L$ and SCr ≥ 1.5 x baseline		**FIRST LINE**	Vancomycin - ORAL [3, 4]	125 mg orally QID for 10-14 days **Children:** 40 mg/kg/day orally divided TID-QID x 10-14 days (Maximum: 2 g/day)	Tablet: $40.00 Diluted IV Sol'n: Varies
			Fidaxomicin [5]	200 mg BID for 10 days	$220.00

Continued ...

C. difficile Infection (CDI)

1) **Prevention: (a) Judicious use of antibiotics.** Receiving an antibiotic, especially clindamycin, extended-spectrum cephalosporin or a fluoroquinolone, is a major risk factor for CDI (Johnston 2007; Owens 2008).

   (b) Use of proton pump inhibitors (PPIs) is independently associated with an increased risk of *C. difficile* (Howell 2010) and administration of PPIs within 14 days of diagnosis of *C. difficile* is an independent risk factor for recurrence (Linsky 2010).

   (c) Diligent hand washing between patient contacts. Note that alcohol and other antiseptics are not effective against *C. difficile* spores. **Meticulous cleaning** of surfaces and equipment with a hospital-grade disinfectant or hypochlorite solution (chlorine bleach).

   (d) Isolation precautions - private rooms or cohorting.

   Clinical Presentation: Symptoms usually begin within 2 weeks, but can start as early as the first day of antibiotic therapy and up to > 6 weeks after therapy has stopped. Usual clinical features include: watery diarrhea (rarely with blood), abdominal cramps/pain, fever, nausea, malaise, anorexia and dehydration. Systemic symptoms are usually absent in mild, but common in moderate-severe disease. Rarely, diarrhea may be absent with severe CDI; this most commonly occurs in postsurgical patients receiving narcotics.

   Diagnosis: Careful history is important with particular emphasis on antibiotic use (past 3 months) and hospitalization. Clinical symptoms plus toxin identification are required.

   Management: Discontinue the precipitating antibiotics, if possible, and administer fluid and electrolytes to maintain hydration. Diarrhea can be expected to resolve in 15-23 % of patients with this approach; for those with mild disease, this may be enough to result in full recovery. If oral antimicrobial therapy is required, metronidazole is preferred in **Mild-Moderate** infection (WBC < 15×10^9/L and SCr < 1.5 times the baseline value); if patient deteriorates or there is an incomplete response by Day 5 of treatment, then change to oral vancomycin and consult infectious disease. If patient cannot tolerate oral therapy, IV metronidazole may be given. In **Severe** infection (WBC ≥ 15×10^9/L or SCr ≥ 1.5 times, admittance to critical care, new elevation in creatinine levels, toxic megacolon, toxic shock), vancomycin should be used initially. **Do not use anti-diarrheals (e.g., loperamide) and opiates as these may precipitate toxic megacolon. Discontinue any laxatives, stool softeners or promotility agents** (Olmos 2007; Pepin 2007).

2) **Treatment of first recurrent CDI** (< 2 months after completion of therapy) typically involves retreatment with the same agent used during initial infection. Metronidazole should not be used beyond the first recurrence or for long-term therapy (Cohen 2010).

3) Vancomycin is administered ORALLY. One option would be to dilute the contents of an intravenous vial (500 mg) into 30 mL of water and then measure the required dose. The patient is permitted to drink this antibiotic solution or the solution may be administered by nasogastric tube (CPS 2012).

4) **Probiotics:** Moderate quality evidence suggests that probiotic prophylaxis in adults and children results in a reduction in *C.difficile* associated diarrhea (CDAD) without an increase in clinically important adverse events (Johnson 2012; Videlock 2012). The results of a few randomized controlled trials suggest that probiotics such as *Lactobacillus spp.* (Beausolil 2007; Gao 2010) and *S. boulardii* (Im 2010; Surawicz 2000) may be helpful in some gastrointestinal disorders, such as CDI and antibiotic-associated diarrhea. While most probiotics have few adverse effects in otherwise healthy people, they have caused serious infections in some highly immunosuppressed or critically ill patients (Med Lettr 2012). Overall, better designed studies are required to define the role of probiotics (Cohen 2010).

5) Fidaxomicin may be considered in patients with severe first episode or recurrent CDI. Significantly fewer patients treated with fidaxomicin vs vancomycin experienced a recurrence of infection; side effects were similar between groups (Cornely 2012; Louis 2011).

References: Bartlett 2009; Beausolil 2007; Bricker 2005; Cloud 2007; Cohen 2010; Cornley 2012; CPS 2012; Crook 2012; Dendukuri 2005; File 2007; Gao 2010; Hawboldt 2005; Hickson 2007, 2011; Howell 2010; Huang 2009; Hyland 2001; Im 2010; Johnston 2007, 2012; Linsky 2010; Louie 2011; McFarland 2006; Med Lettr 2012; Nelson 2007; Pepin 2007; Pillai 2008; Poutanen 2004; Schroeder 2005; Shen 2007; Simor 2004, 2010; Surawicz 2000, 2008; Videlock 2012.

Modifying Circumstances		Antibiotic Choice(s)	Usual Dosage	Cost per Week

Malaria Prophylaxis - Adult & Children [1, 2]

Modifying Circumstances		Antibiotic Choice(s)	Usual Dosage	Cost per Week
CHLOROQUINE SENSITIVE Includes: Central America (except Panama) Mexico, Argentina, Paraguay, Northern Africa, states of the former Soviet Union, parts of China and the Middle East, Caribbean (**NOT travellers to resorts**).	*FIRST LINE*	Chloroquine phosphate [3] 250 mg (~150 mg base) per tablet	500 mg (300 mg base) once per week **Children:** 8 mg/kg (5 mg/kg base) once per week up to maximum 300 mg base	$0.64
	ALTERNATIVE	Mefloquine [3, 4]	Loading dose of 250 mg base (1 tab) daily for 3 days, then one 250 mg tab per week **Children: see page 107.**	$3.57
		Doxycycline [4]	100 mg once daily **Children > 8 years OR > 25 kg:** see page 107.	$4.10
		Atovaquone-Proguanil [4] (MALARONE, MALARONE PEDIATRIC)	250 mg/100 mg (1 Malarone tablet) once daily **Children: see page 107.**	$36.54
CHLOROQUINE RESISTANT (MEFLOQUINE SENSITIVE) Sub-Sahara Africa, South America (except Argentina and Paraguay), Oceania, Asia	*FIRST LINE*	Mefloquine [3, 4] (LARIAM)	250 mg base once per week **Children: see page 107.**	$3.57
		Atovaquone-Proguanil [4] (MALARONE, MALARONE PEDIATRIC)	250 mg/100 mg (1 Malarone tablet) once daily **Children: see page 107.**	$36.54
		Doxycycline [4]	100 mg once daily **Children > 8 years OR > 25 kg:** see page 107.	$4.10
	ALTERNATIVE	Primaquine phosphate [4, 5] 26.3 mg (15 mg base) per tablet	30 mg base daily (2 tabs) **Children (> 9 years old):** 0.5 mg base/kg daily (Maximum: 30 mg)	$5.37
CHLOROQUINE AND MEFLOQUINE RESISTANT OR CONTRA-INDICATED Thai-Cambodian and Thai-Myanmar borders, Eastern Myanmar, Western Cambodia, and South/Central Vietnam	*FIRST LINE*	Doxycycline [4]	100 mg once daily **Children: see page 107.**	$4.10
		Atvaquone-Proguanil [4] (MALARONE, MALARONE PEDIATRIC)	250 mg/100 mg (1 Malarone tablet) once daily **Children: see page 107.**	$36.54

Malaria Prophylaxis - Dosing in Children

Mefloquine	Doxycycline	Atovaquone-Proguanil

Mefloquine	Doxycycline	Atovaquone-Proguanil (as single daily dose)		
5–9 kg: 1/8 tablet per week or 31.25 mg base per week	> 8 years = 2 mg/kg/day	**Weight**	**Malarone Pediatric** (62.5/25 mg)	**Malarone** (250/100 mg)
10–19 kg: 1/4 tablet per week	25-35 kg or 8-10 years: 50 mg	5-8 kg	½ tablet	------
20–29 kg: 1/2 tablet per week	36-50 kg or 11-13 years: 75 mg	9-10 kg	¾ tablet	------
30–45 kg: 3/4 tablet per week	> 50 kg or ≥ 14 years: 100 mg	11-20 kg	1 tablet	¼ tablet
> 45 kg: 1 tablet per week	(Maximum: 100 mg/day)	21-30 kg	2 tablets	½ tablet
		31-40 kg	3 tablets	¾ tablet
		> 40 kg	-------	1 tablet

1) Recommendations for malaria prophylaxis and list of travel medicine clinics in Canada: www. travelhealth.gc.ca or www.cdc.gov. The WHO International travel website also provides a search by country for resistance patterns and recommended prophylaxis: www.who.int. When determining if prophylaxis is important, consider malaria endemicity, season, altitude, degree of rural travel, age, pregnancy, allergies and concurrent medications/illnesses. All travellers to an endemic area require prophylaxis and protective measures, such as use of DEET insect repellents and insecticide treated bed nets. Insect repellents containing a maximum of 35% DEET (30% if extended duration product) should be applied, especially after dusk; higher concentrations of DEET offer no additional advantage. DEET is safe for use in pregnant and breast-feeding women. Lower concentrations of DEET are recommended for children; the American Academy of Pediatrics (2008) recommends 30% DEET down to 2 month of age. An alternative is lemon eucalyptus oil. Advise travellers to buy their full supply of medications before departure as the sale of counterfeit antimalarials is widespread in the developing world (Dondorp 2004).

2) The duration of chemoprophylaxis is as follows (CATMAT 2009; Suh 2004):

   Atovaquone-proguanil: starting 1 day before entering malaria-endemic region, daily during exposure and for 1 week after departure. Administer with meal.

   Chloroquine: starting 1-2 weeks before entering malaria-endemic region, weekly during exposure and for 4 weeks after departure.

   Doxycycline: starting 1 day before entering malaria-endemic region, daily during exposure and for 4 weeks after departure.

   Mefloquine: starting 1-3 weeks before entering malaria-endemic region, weekly during exposure and for 4 weeks after departure. Administer with meal and at least 240 mL of water.

   Primaquine: starting 1 day before entering malaria-endemic region, daily during exposure and for 3 days after departure. Administer with food.

   If fever develops within one year, and particularly within three months of returning, the patient should be considered to have malaria, regardless of prevention. Investigate urgently using thick and thin blood films or a rapid diagnostic test to rule out malaria. If negative, repeat them twice over 48 hours (Wobeser 2011).

3) Hydroxychloroquine is an acceptable alternative to chloroquine: Children: 6.5 mg/kg (5 mg/kg base) once per week up to maximum 400 mg (310 mg base) once per week; Adults: 400 mg (310 mg base) once per week. Start 1-2 weeks before travelling and continue weekly x 4 weeks after departure.
   Chloroquine is contraindicated in generalized psoriasis and seizure disorder (Suh 2004).
   Mefloquine should not be prescribed for prophylaxis in patients with active depression, a recent history of depression, generalized anxiety disorder, psychosis, or schizophrenia or other major psychiatric disorders, or with a history of convulsions or cardiac conductive disturbances.

4) Use in pregnancy: Mefloquine should be avoided in the 1st trimester and advise women to avoid pregnancy within 3 months of stopping prophylaxis; it can be used with caution in the 2nd and 3rd trimesters. Doxycycline is contraindicated in pregnancy, during breast feeding and in children < 8 years. Atovaquone-Proguanil (Malarone) and primaquine are contraindicated in pregnancy (Suh 2004).

5) G6PD level must be normal. Check G6PD level before initiating therapy. Take with food.

References: Am Acad Ped 2008; Baird 2003; Boggild 2007; Bradley 2003; CATMAT 2009; CCDR 2004; CDC 2008; Chen 2005, 2006, 2010; Chiodini 2007; Cot 2003; Dondorp 2004; FDA Med Watch 2002; Hill 2006; Koren 2003; Suh 2004; WHO 2008; Wobeser 2011.

© 2013 Anti-infective Review Panel

‡ Common oral dosage ranges are provided unless otherwise stated. Consult the drug monograph for details on age and condition-specific dosing. **Page 107**

Prevention of Infective Endocarditis [1, 2]

DENTAL AND UPPER RESPIRATORY PROCEDURES [2]	**FIRST LINE**	**Amoxicillin**	2 g given 30-60 minutes pre-procedure **Children:** 50 mg/kg
	SECOND LINE	**Cephalexin**	2 g given 30-60 minutes pre-procedure **Children:** 50 mg/kg
		Cefadroxil	2 g given 30-60 minutes pre-procedure
		Clindamycin	600mg given 30-60 minutes pre-procedure **Children:** 20 mg/kg
		Azithromycin	500 mg given 30-60 minutes pre-procedure **Children:** 10 mg/kg
		Clarithromycin	500 mg given 30-60 minutes pre-procedure Children: 15 mg/kg
PARENTERAL [2]	**FIRST LINE**	**Ampicillin**	2 g IM [3] or IV given 30-60 minutes pre-procedure **Children:** 50 mg/kg IM or IV
		Cefazolin	1 g IM [3] or IV given 30-60 minutes pre-procedure **Children:** 50 mg/kg IM or IV
		Clindamycin	600 mg IV given 30-60 minutes pre-procedure **Children:** 20 mg/kg IV
GI AND GU PROCEDURES			Antibiotic prophylaxis solely to prevent IE is no longer routinely recommended for genitourinary (GU) and gastrointestinal (GI) procedures.

1) **Prophylaxis is recommended ONLY for the following;**
   Cardiac conditions associated with the highest risk of adverse outcomes from endocarditis; except for these conditions, antibiotic prophylaxis is no longer recommended for any other congenital heart disease:
   Prosthetic heart valves or prosthetic material used for cardiac repair
   Previous bacterial endocarditis (even in the absence of heart disease)
   Unrepaired cyanotic congenital heart disease (includes palliative shunts and conduits)
   During the first 6 months after complete repair of a congenital heart defect with prosthetic materials/device
   Repaired congenital heart disease with residual defects that inhibit endothelialization
   Cardiac transplant recipients who develop cardiac valvulopathy
   Dental: All dental procedures that involve manipulation of gingival tissue of the periapical region of teeth or perforation of the oral mucosa.
   Respiratory: Tonsillectomy or adenoidectomy, surgical operations involving respiratory mucosa, bronchoscopy, invasive treatment of established infection.
   Skin: Antibiotic prophylaxis is reasonable for procedures on infected skin, skin structures, or musculoskeletal tissue only for high risk patients listed above.
   Genitourinary or GI: Prophylaxis not routinely recommended. Cytoscopy or other urinary tract manipulations on patients who have an enterococcal UTI or colonization.
2) Oral regimens are more convenient and safer. Parenteral regimens if unable to take/absorb oral medications.
3) IM administration should be avoided in patients receiving anticoagulation therapy.

References: Allen 2010; Dajani 1997; Desime 2012; Duval 2012; Gould 2006; Horstkotte 2004; NICE 2008; Nishimura 2008; Sroussi 2007; Wieler 1999; Wilson (AHA) 2007, 2008.

Extended Interval Aminoglycoside Dosing Method

Rationale

- Aminoglycosides are conventionally administered in divided doses over a 24 hour period to target specific peak/trough serum concentrations. For extended interval aminoglycoside dosing a single dose is given in a 24 hour or longer period. This dosing method maximizes the peak concentration/ MIC ratio and takes advantage of the concentration-dependent bactericidal effect of aminoglycosides.
- Aminoglycosides can be given at an extended interval without compromising therapeutic efficacy or safety. The risk of nephrotoxicity compared to conventional dosing is equal or less and the risk for ototoxicity is comparable.
- All aminoglycosides may cause or increase neuromuscular blockade. Use with caution in patients with neuromuscular disorders, including myasthenia gravis. Aminoglycosides also display a post-antibiotic effect where bacterial growth is inhibited despite drug levels being undetectable.

Contraindications to Using Extended Interval Aminoglycoside Dosing		
• Neonates	• Osteomyelitis	• Burn patients with >20% of body surface area
• Pregnancy	• Meningitis	• Renal impairment (CrCl < 40 mL/min)
• Endocarditis	• Dialysis	• Septic shock (during initial hemodynamic instability)
• Febrile neutropenia	• Surgical prophylaxis	
• Ascites	• Cystic fibrosis	• Synergistic therapy (i.e. beta-lactam + aminoglycoside for enterococcal infection)

Adult Dosage Guidelines

Dose and dosing interval (e.g., gentamicin 250 mg q24h) can be calculated using two steps:

STEP #1: Calculate Dose (mg/kg) based on Ideal Body Weight (IBW)

Drug and Dose	Rounding of dose:
Gentamicin or **tobramycin**: 5 - 7 mg/kg **Amikacin**: 15 mg/kg	Varies with local hospital practices

Dose is based upon Ideal Body Weight (IBW) in kg

IBW Males:	50 kg + (2.3 x inches over 5 feet)
IBW Females:	45.5 kg + (2.3 x inches over 5 feet)
Obesity:	(Actual body weight > 25-30% of calculated IBW): use IBW + 0.4 (Actual BW-IBW) If actual body weight (ABW) < IBW, use ABW in creatinine clearance calculation

STEP #2: Determine Dosing Interval Based on Creatinine Clearance

Estimated Creatinine Clearance

Male: Estimated CrCl (mL/min) = $\dfrac{(140 - age) \times Weight\ (Kg)}{Serum\ creatinine\ (\mu mol/L)} \times 1.2$

Female: Estimated CrCl = [same equation as above for male] x 0.85

Conversions

1 inch	=	2.54 cm
12 inches	=	1 foot
1 kg	=	2.2 lbs
88.4 µmol/L	=	1 mg/dL

Creatinine Clearance (mL/min)	Dosing Interval
≥ 60	q24h
40-59	q36h
< 40	Avoid extended interval dosing and consider conventional dosing

Continued...

Extended Interval Aminoglycoside Dosing Method

Monitoring

Parameter	Frequency
Serum creatinine	• Before starting therapy • 2-3 times weekly • If serum creatinine rises by ≥ 25% from baseline, reconsider use of aminoglycoside
Levels	• Standard peak levels are not indicated • Consider trough (0-60 minutes prior to dose) levels: 　- Receiving > 3-5 days of therapy; 　- Suspected changes in renal clearance; 　- Changes in volume of distribution; 　- Concomitant use of nephrotoxic drugs; 　- Elderly patients 　- Severe infection • Trough level should be measured at least once weekly for a desired level < 0.5-1 mcg/mL • Measure trough level more frequently (e.g., every 3 days) when there is a significant change in renal function (e.g., ≥ 25% change), if the patient has renal dysfunction or if they are on concurrent nephrotoxic drugs • If level is greater than desired trough, extend dosing interval by 12 hours and repeat level prior to next dose. If the next level continues to be high, then change to conventional dosing method
Symptoms of ototoxicity	• Monitor for cochlear (e.g., tinnitus, loss of hearing, sense of fullness in ears) and vestibular toxicity (e.g., loss of balance, oscillopsia) before starting therapy then daily • Risk factors for ototoxicity (cochlear or vestibulotoxicity) include: Treatment >14 days with a total cumulative dosage > 2.5 g; concomitant renal impairment; concomitant use of other ototoxic medications (e.g., loop diuretics, antineoplastic agents, vancomycin); and past history of ototoxicity.

References: Anaizi 1997; Baily 1997; Ferrois-Lisart 1996; Freemen 1997; Munckhof 1996; Nicolau 1995; Schumock 1995; Traynor 1995, 1995; Urban 1999; Uijtendaal 2001; Miron 2001; Tiwari 2009.

Comment Sheet

We welcome your participation in the revision to the guidelines by receiving your comments on how to improve them. You may also submit an online form which is available at:

www.mumshealth.com/content/order_forms/guideline_comment_sheet.pdf

Item	Comments
1. Is this guideline concise, easy to understand? ❑ Yes ❑ No	
2. Would you recommend any content changes or new topic additions? ❑ Yes ❑ No	
3. Would you recommend any format changes? ❑ Yes ❑ No	
4. How often do you refer to guidelines in your practice? ❑ **Daily** ❑ **Weekly** ❑ **Monthly** ❑ **Rarely**	

To assure accurate acknowledgment in the guidelines as an external reviewer, please provide the following information:

Name: _____ Type of Practice: _____

Affiliation (if applicable): _____

City/Town: _____ Province: _____

Phone: _____ Fax: _____ Email: _____

Please return to:

MUMS Guideline Clearinghouse - www.mumshealth.com
Suite 200 – 301 Donlands Ave., Toronto, ON M4J 3R8
fax (416) 597-8574 (toll-free: 1-866-540-1847) or e-mail: guidelines@mumshealth.com

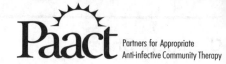

Paact
Partners for Appropriate
Anti-infective Community Therapy

The PAACT (PArtners for Appropriate Community Therapy) MAINPRO-C® CME program was initially developed by a group of family physicians and pharmacists in the mid 1990s in order to help integrate the Anti-infective Guideline recommendations into practice. PAACT has been evaluated extensively and is up-dated on an on-going basis.

It can play a pivotal role in a community-based antimicrobial stewardship program

This interactive program consists of front-line cases that are designed to highlight common, office-based scenarios. The case studies combined with the guidelines form the basis for interdisciplinary, local sessions. These programs are accredited by the College of Family Physicians of Canada.

If you are interested in running a program in your community, please fill in the information below in order to provide more details and a cost estimate.

DESCRIPTION (These sessions may be run over half-days and/or as lunch and learn - See website for program details)	Check program of interest	Number of participants	Facilitator(s) Required
PAACT Anti-infective Program (12 Credit Program)			Yes / No
PAACT Anemia Program (5 credit Program)			Yes / No
PAACT Hypertension Program (4 Credit Program)			Yes / No
PAACT Respiratory Program (5 Credit Program)			Yes / No
Each Program INCLUDES: **Facilitator Manual** **Participant Manuals** **Supplemental materials (e.g., non-Rx pads)** **Guidelines (if needed)** **Evaluation forms (on-site and post-reflective if facilitated small group)** **Certificate - Post program**			

Name: _____		**Street Address:** _____	
Phone: _____			
Fax: _____		**City/Province:** _____	
E-mail: _____		**Postal Code:** _____	
Possible Dates: _____			

1. Stewart J, Pilla J, Dunn L. Pilot study for appropriate anti-infective community therapy. Can Fam Phys 2000;46:851-9.
2. Juzych NS, Banerjee M, Essenmacher L, Lerner SA. Improvements in antimicrobial prescribing for treatment of upper respiratory tract infections through provider education. J Gen Intern Med 2005;20:901–5.

paact@mumshealth.com   www.paact.org
Tel: (416) 597-6867; 1-877-876-4580   Fax: (416) 597-8574; 1-866-540-1847